VITAMIN E

**Everything
You Need
to Know**

Other Books From the People's Medical Society

Alzheimer's and Dementia: Questions You Have . . . Answers You Need

Arthritis: Questions You Have . . . Answers You Need

Asthma: Questions You Have . . . Answers You Need

Cholesterol and Triglycerides: Questions You Have . . . Answers You Need

Diabetes: Questions You Have . . . Answers You Need

Prostate: Questions You Have . . . Answers You Need

Stroke: Questions You Have . . . Answers You Need

Vitamin C: Everything You Need to Know

Vitamins and Minerals: Questions You Have . . . Answers You Need

Your Eyes: Questions You Have . . . Answers You Need

Your Heart: Questions You Have . . . Answers You Need

VITAMIN E

Everything You Need to Know

By Jennifer Hay

≣People's Medical Society®

Allentown, Pennsylvania

The People's Medical Society is a nonprofit consumer health organization dedicated to the principles of better, more responsive and less expensive medical care. Organized in 1983, the People's Medical Society puts previously unavailable medical information into the hands of consumers so that they can make informed decisions about their own health care.

Membership in the People's Medical Society is $20 a year and includes a subscription to the *People's Medical Society Newsletter.* For information, write to the People's Medical Society, 462 Walnut Street, Allentown, PA 18102, or call 610-770-1670.

This and other People's Medical Society publications are available for quantity purchase at discount. Contact the People's Medical Society for details.

Many of the designations used by manufacturers and sellers to distinguish their products are claimed as trademarks. Where those designations appear in this book and the People's Medical Society was aware of a trademark claim, the designations have been printed in initial capital letters (e.g., Deprenyl).

© 1998 by the People's Medical Society
Printed in the United States of America

All rights reserved. No part of this publication may be reproduced or transmitted in any form or by any means, electronic or mechanical, including photocopy, recording or any information storage and retrieval system, without the written permission of the publisher.

Library of Congress Cataloging-in-Publication Data
Hay, Jennifer, 1964–
    Vitamin E : everything you need to know / by Jennifer Hay.
      p. cm.
    Includes index.
    ISBN 1-882606-37-X
    1. Vitamin E—Miscellanea.   2. Vitamin E—Physiological effect.
I. Title.
QP772.T6H39   1998
612.3'99—dc21   98-10812
                                                                          CIP

1 2 3 4 5 6 7 8 9 0
First printing, April 1998

CONTENTS

Introduction 7

Chapter 1 The Basics 11

Chapter 2 Vitamin E and Its Uses 21
       Vitamin E and the Cardiovascular System 24
         Vitamin E and Atherosclerosis 29
           Vitamin E and Cholesterol 32
           Vitamin E and White Blood Cells 36
           Vitamin E and Smooth Muscle Cells 37
           Vitamin E and Blood Vessels 37
           Vitamin E and the Blood 39
         Vitamin E and Blood Flow 41
         Vitamin E and Heart Disease 43
         Vitamin E and Stroke 46
       Vitamin E and the Immune System 49
         Vitamin E and Immune Response 50
         Vitamin E and Cancer 56
           Vitamin E and Cancer Risk 57
           Vitamin E and Cancer Treatment 63
       Vitamin E and the Nervous System 65

　　　　　　Vitamin E and the Respiratory System 72
　　　　　　Vitamin E and the Eyes 75
　　　　　　Vitamin E and the Skin 78
　　　　　　Vitamin E and Diabetes 81
　　　　　　Other Vitamin E Uses 84
　　　　　　　　Vitamin E and Muscle Function 84
　　　　　　　　Vitamin E and Women's Health 86
　　　　　　　　Vitamin E and Rheumatoid Arthritis 87
　　　　　　　　Vitamin E and Liver Function 87
　　　　　　　　Vitamin E and Fertility 88
　　　　　　Putting It All Together 89

Chapter 3 **What Else Do I Need to Know?** 93
　　　　　　Dosage 93
　　　　　　Toxicity 100
　　　　　　Drug Interactions 101
　　　　　　Nutrient Interactions 102
　　　　　　Supplements 103
　　　　　　Dietary Sources 109

Glossary 113

Index 121

INTRODUCTION

About 40 years ago, when I was a kid growing up in Chicago, I remember riding in a car to a Chicago Cubs game with one of my best friends and our fathers. My friend and I were in the backseat strategizing what seats in Wrigley Field would afford us the best chance of nabbing a foul ball. In the front seat, our fathers were having their own discussion, and it wasn't about baseball.

My friend's dad was telling my father about vitamin E. That's right—vitamin E. It seems he had been doing some reading, and as a result, he had become a strong believer in taking vitamin E supplements. The reason I remember their conversation is because it struck me as being odd. I had never heard anyone talking about vitamins and minerals, other than my mother when she was sticking that spoonful of liquid vitamins into my mouth during my prekindergarten years. But here were two grown, actually middle-aged, men talking about vitamin E. And to be honest, I had never heard of vitamin E before.

My friend's father was saying that he was taking vitamin E to protect his heart. Both his parents and several of his aunts and uncles had died of heart disease before they were 55 years old. He was nearing 50 himself and was worried that he, too, might be a victim. He figured that if these new findings about vitamin E were correct, he would extend his life.

For a kid not even a teenager yet, I was very taken by his comments. Could vitamins be that important? Could taking a vitamin E supplement really make a difference in his life?

Since then, I've paid a lot of attention to vitamins and minerals, especially vitamin E. And over the years more, and better, information about the importance of vitamin E has come to light. Each year there are new studies and reports telling us how vitamin E helps prevent certain medical conditions. Plus, we are learning how it might be useful in treating conditions such as Alzheimer's disease. While not necessarily a "wonder" vitamin, it is certainly becoming a more important one.

It's because of that importance that we have produced this book. With all the news and information coming out about vitamin E, we felt it was time that all the best information be put in one place. And the pages that follow are that place. Author Jennifer Hay reports everything you need to know about vitamin E. In an easy-to-read, question-and-answer format, she guides you through the hype and the truth.

Our goal at the People's Medical Society is to empower you with the information and knowledge you need to make sound medical decisions. This book is a major step in that direction for it presents, in a clear and understandable way, everything you need to know about one of today's hottest health topics.

And, oh, by the way: My friend's father has been taking vitamin E supplements for more than 40 years now. Next year, he will celebrate his 90th birthday!

CHARLES B. INLANDER
President
People's Medical Society

VITAMIN E

Everything You Need to Know

Terms printed in boldface can be found in the glossary, beginning on page 113. Only the first mention of the word in the text will be boldfaced.

We have tried to use male and female pronouns in an egalitarian manner throughout the book. Any imbalance in usage has been in the interest of readability.

1 THE BASICS

Q: What is **vitamin E**?

A: Vitamin E, a light yellow oil that comes in a variety of forms, is one of the most commonly supplemented **nutrients** in the United States; it is second only to vitamin C in popularity, and its popularity is on the rise. Sales of vitamin E **supplements** have been increasing at a rate of 10 percent annually in recent years.

Q: Why is that?

A: Primarily because researchers have linked vitamin E to a variety of health benefits, including the prevention or slowing of heart disease, Alzheimer's disease and cancer.

Q: I want to know all about this research. But first, I need to know a little more about vitamin E itself. You said it comes in a variety of forms?

A: Yes. In fact, "vitamin E" is a generic term that refers to any of eight separate compounds that exhibit vitamin E activity. These compounds come in two classes—**tocopherols**

and **tocotrienols**—and vary significantly in potency. The most active form is **alpha-tocopherol**. In fact, vitamin E is often referred to as alpha-tocopherol or simply tocopherol.

Q: What else can you tell me about vitamin E?

A: Vitamin E is **fat soluble**, which means that it requires a little bit of fat for absorption. This also means that excess amounts can be stored in the body—generally in fatty tissue, muscle and the liver.

Q: Aren't all vitamins stored in the body?

A: No. Excess amounts of **water-soluble** vitamins, such as vitamin C and the B vitamins, are eliminated from the body.

Q: What does vitamin E do in the body?

A: While vitamin E may have a variety of functions, to date researchers have identified only one primary function—it acts as an **antioxidant**.

> "Vitamin E is the most effective chain-breaking lipid-soluble antioxidant in the biological membrane, where it contributes to membrane stability. It protects critical cellular structures against damage from oxygen-free radicals . . . and reactive products of lipid peroxidation."
> —Mohsen Meydani, Ph.D.
> *Lancet*, January 21, 1995

Q: What is an antioxidant?

A: An antioxidant is a substance that inhibits oxidative reactions.

Q: I don't really understand that definition. Could you explain further?

A: Certainly. To understand what an antioxidant is, you need to know a little bit about **oxidation**, a chemical process in which a molecule combines with oxygen and loses electrons.

You may recall from chemistry class that atoms contain a nucleus of protons and neutrons surrounded by electrons. These negatively charged electrons generally move in pairs. Occasionally, however, an atom or molecule contains one or more unpaired electrons. These "lone wolf" particles, known as **free radicals**, make the atom or molecule reactive. Atoms or molecules containing free radicals attempt to steal electrons from other atoms or molecules to retain their balance. Those atoms or molecules victimized by free radicals themselves become free radicals, initiating a chain reaction of multiplying free radicals.

Q: What do these free radicals do?

A: Free radicals can destroy enzymes, protein molecules and cells. They can interfere with a cell's ability to take in nutrients and expel waste, affecting its ability to perform its functions. They can damage a cell's genetic material—its DNA—causing mutations that may have the potential to lead to cancer. And they can damage fat compounds in the body, causing them to turn rancid and release more free radicals. This process, known as **lipid peroxidation**, is thought to play a role in cardiovascular disease. In fact, free radicals have been implicated in a variety of diseases as well as the aging process.

Q: You said these free radicals are created when molecules combine with oxygen. When does this occur?

A: Oxidative reactions take place in our bodies all the time. We use oxygen for a variety of cellular activities—from generating energy to manufacturing enzymes. The very cellular activities that keep us alive involve oxidation and the production of free radicals. In fact, cells in our **immune system** deliberately make free radicals to kill bacteria, viruses and other harmful foreign organisms.

Exposure to substances in our environment—ultraviolet light, tobacco smoke and pollutants, for example—can also trigger the production of free radicals.

Q: OK. I think I've got the idea. Now could you tell me again where antioxidants fit in?

A: Antioxidants donate electrons to free radicals, thus neutralizing them. This gesture stops the free radical chain reaction and renders the antioxidant inactive.

Q: How does all this relate to vitamin E?

A: Vitamin E, as we've said, is an antioxidant. It has been shown to stop oxidative reactions. Many researchers theorize that vitamin E and other antioxidant nutrients may help protect us from damage caused by free radicals, which, as we've said, have been implicated in a number of diseases.

Q: But what, specifically, does vitamin E do?

A: Vitamin E's antioxidant abilities enable it to protect cells and membranes against free radical damage, thus stabilizing the membranes, and to protect fats in the body—notably polyunsaturated fats—from oxidation. It also helps protect the lungs against oxidative damage from air pollutants and protects the tissues of the skin, eyes, liver, breasts and calf muscles.

Q: **That's a pretty impressive assortment of duties. Do other antioxidants do the same things?**

A: Some perform similar functions. For example, vitamin C, like vitamin E, is known to protect the lungs, skin and eyes from oxidative damage. But vitamin C and other antioxidant nutrients also perform functions that vitamin E doesn't; for example, vitamin C has been shown in some studies to restore vitamin E to its potent antioxidant state after vitamin E has been rendered inactive by neutralizing free radicals. It takes all of the antioxidant nutrients working together to provide protection throughout the body.

Q: **What other nutrients act as antioxidants?**

A: In addition to vitamins E and C, the antioxidant nutrients include beta carotene and the **mineral** selenium.

Q: **I have a general understanding of what vitamins and minerals are, but I don't really know the difference between them. What are the basic definitions?**

A: Vitamins and minerals are nutrients—food components obtained from our diets—that have been found to be essential in small quantities for human life. Vitamins are organic compounds; this means that they contain carbon and come from living materials—plants or animals—or from substances derived from living materials, such as petroleum products.

Minerals, in contrast, are inorganic compounds; they do not contain carbon and do not originate from living organisms.

Q: That clears things up for me. Getting back to vitamin E, does it have any other functions?

A: Vitamin E appears to be necessary for normal functioning of the nervous and reproductive systems, for muscle development and for making and maintaining red blood cells, which carry oxygen to tissues throughout the body.

Q: You say "appears to be necessary." What's the scoop?

A: Researchers have not yet pinpointed exactly what role vitamin E plays in these functions. They do know, however, that problems arise in these areas when vitamin E is deficient.

Q: That reminds me. What are the signs of vitamin E deficiency?

A: The classic symptoms include **anemia**, which is caused by the premature aging and death of red blood cells; hemorrhage, or bleeding; and neurological disturbances such as inability to concentrate, loss of balance and a staggering gait.

Q: Do many people develop these symptoms?

A: No. Most people do not develop vitamin E deficiency symptoms. Remember: Vitamin E is fat soluble; it can be stored in the body, so it's possible to take in less than what is needed and still remain healthy.

People who do not absorb fat normally; premature, very low birth weight infants; older people; people on very low-fat diets; and people with chronic liver disease or **cystic fibrosis** are at higher risk of developing a vitamin E deficiency, however.

Q: How much vitamin E do we need?

A: The **Recommended Dietary Allowance (RDA)**, the amount that the National Academy of Sciences' Food and Nutrition Board considers to be adequate to meet the known nutrient needs of most healthy individuals, is 15 **international units (I.U.)**, 10 **tocopherol equivalents (TE)**, or 10 milligrams TE for men, and 12 I.U., 8 TE or 8 milligrams TE for women.

Q: Whoa. What kind of measurements are those?

A: International units and tocopherol equivalents are arbitrary measurements that take into consideration the potencies of the various forms of vitamin E so that the forms can be compared with one another. However, the two forms of measurements cannot be compared with one another.

Q: Why? What's the difference between the two measurements?

A: The international unit is used as a measure for both vitamin E and vitamin A. The tocopherol equivalent, as its name implies, is used solely to measure vitamin E.

Q: How does this all break down in terms of a measurement I can relate to?

A: One I.U. of vitamin E is equal to 1 milligram of synthetic alpha-tocopherol. One milligram TE, or 1 TE, is equal to 1.49 I.U. of natural alpha-tocopherol.

Q: I thought I read somewhere that the RDA is 30 I.U. Did it change?

A: Not exactly, although it might in the future. The 30 I.U. recommendation you saw is called a **Reference Daily Intake (RDI)**, or **Daily Value**. It's the figure the U.S. Food and Drug Administration mandates be used on food labels. The term RDI recently replaced old U.S. RDAs; they are derived from the RDAs set by the National Academy of Sciences and are usually similar. In the case of vitamin E, however, the RDI is higher than the RDA.

Q: I think I understand. But didn't you just say that the RDAs themselves may soon change?

A: Yes. The Food and Nutrition Board is in the process of reviewing, updating and actually replacing the RDAs with what are known as **Dietary Reference Intakes**, or **DRIs**. These guidelines, which will be introduced sporadically from now through the year 2000, place more emphasis on the benefits people can derive from nutrients than do the existing RDAs.

Q: In what way?

A: The DRIs include revised RDAs designed not only to prevent deficiency diseases but also to decrease the risk of chronic diseases such as cancer, heart disease and osteoporosis. The revised RDAs are based on the Estimated Average Requirement, the intake that meets the estimated nutrient need of half the individuals in a specific group. If not enough information is available to determine an average requirement, the DRIs include an Adequate Intake, an amount shown by experimental or observational data to sustain a specific indicator of health, such as calcium retention in bone. Finally, the DRIs include a Tolerable Upper Intake Level, the maximum amount of a nutrient unlikely to cause side effects in most healthy people.

Q: Will the DRI indicate a higher intake of vitamin E?

A: That remains to be seen; however, many of the recent studies that have shown health benefits from vitamin E have involved doses of 100 I.U. or more—well above the current RDA.

Q: Is there any proof that these larger doses could be harmful?

A: For the most part, vitamin E is considered to be quite safe, even in large amounts. Very high doses—more than 1,200 I.U. per day—have been reported to cause nausea, flatulence, diarrhea, headache, heart palpitations and fainting. These symptoms disappear when the dosage is reduced.

Q: Anything else?

A: In terms of symptoms, no. But people who are taking **anticoagulant** drugs such as warfarin should avoid high doses of vitamin E since the vitamin itself has anticoagulant effects.

Q: Are high doses easy to get from foods?

A: No. In fact, many people do not even get the RDA from the foods they eat.

Q: In what foods is vitamin E found?

A: The richest dietary sources include wheat germ; soybean, cotton seed, peanut, corn, hazelnut, sunflower and almond oils; whole grain cereals; eggs; mayonnaise; and whole, raw seeds and nuts. Fortified cereals, too, provide a decent amount.

Q: No wonder people have trouble getting enough! Most of those foods are not foods people eat in abundance. Where do we get most of our vitamin E?

A: According to one study, people are most likely to get their vitamin E from mayonnaise and salad dressings; margarine; doughnuts, cookies and cakes; french fries and fried potatoes; salad and cooking oils; pies; and eggs.

Q: Do people get enough vitamin E?

A: Although deficiency symptoms are rare, studies show that many people do not take in the RDA. And it's virtually impossible to get the large doses of vitamin E shown in clinical trials to be beneficial through diet. But, as we've said, vitamin E supplements are becoming increasingly popular as new research uncovers potential health benefits. We discuss this research in the next chapter.

2 VITAMIN E AND ITS USES

Q: You said in chapter 1 that vitamin E has been linked to a number of health benefits. What are they?

A: The benefit that has gotten the most press in recent years is vitamin E's apparent ability to protect the heart and blood vessels. A number of studies have shown that people who take in enough vitamin E have a reduced risk of heart disease and **stroke**. But that's not vitamin E's only claim to fame. It has also been credited with the following:

- improving **immune response**

- protecting against cancer

- slowing the progression of neurological problems such as **Alzheimer's disease**

- protecting the lungs

- protecting against **cataracts**

- decreasing the complications of **diabetes**

- reducing muscle soreness

Q: Can vitamin E really do all that?

A: Maybe, maybe not. Many of the claims made for vitamin E have some substance; they are rooted in scientific theory and supported, at least in part, by research. But the research often conflicts. One well-designed study may show that vitamin E provides a substantial health benefit; the next study on the very same subject may show that it has no effect or even a negative effect. Clearly, more research is needed. Until a consensus emerges, vitamin E's various health benefits remain a matter of speculation.

Q: Is there any chance that vitamin E may do at least some of what it's claimed to do?

A: Yes. The evidence available thus far indicates that vitamin E may indeed play a role in helping our bodies fight disease. In fact, support for vitamin E's ability to protect the heart is now strong enough that many doctors recommend vitamin E to their patients—and/or take it themselves.

Q: Really?

A: Really. Nearly two-thirds of heart specialists attending a 1994 conference sponsored by the American College of Cardiology indicated that they take antioxidant vitamins daily. When they were asked why, a number pointed to recent studies linking vitamin E to lower risk of heart disease and said that while there is no definitive proof of a link, the vitamin E therapy can't hurt, could help and is inexpensive (*Internal Medicine News,* March 1, 1994).

Primary-care physicians apparently share this viewpoint. Editorials for and against antioxidant supplements that appeared in a 1996 issue of *Medical Tribune* sparked numerous calls to the newspaper's hotline. And nine out of 10 of the doctors who responded endorsed the role of antioxidants—including vitamin E—in fighting disease. As one doctor told the paper, "Antioxidants are relatively inexpensive, completely safe in recommended doses and, as health insurance goes, a genuine bargain" (*Medical Tribune,* March 21, 1996).

Q: That's some pretty strong support! What's the basis for it?

A: In recent years, researchers have been looking into the possibility that antioxidants may help prevent the degenerative diseases of aging, and some **epidemiologic studies** have linked low intakes or low blood levels of antioxidant nutrients such as vitamin E with increased mortality from chronic diseases.

Q: Wait a minute. Why are researchers looking at both intake and blood levels? Doesn't a low intake automatically result in a low blood level and a high intake automatically result in a high blood level?

A: In most cases yes, but blood or **plasma** levels of vitamin E—and other nutrients, for that matter—are also affected by a variety of other factors such as illness and a person's ability to absorb the vitamin. For example, as we said in chapter 1, people who have difficulty absorbing fats and people with chronic liver disease or cystic fibrosis may have difficulty absorbing vitamin E and may develop deficiencies.

Q: OK. Getting back to those studies that link vitamin E intake or blood levels with mortality from chronic diseases. Could you give me an example of what they show?

A: Certainly. Researchers at the National Institute on Aging compared the use of vitamin E and vitamin C supplements with the death rates in 11,179 seniors during a three-year period and found that those who used both supplements were 42 percent less likely to die of any cause and 53 percent less likely to die of heart problems during the period than were those who used neither supplement.

Those who used vitamin E alone were 34 percent less likely to die of any cause and 47 percent less likely to die of heart problems during the period. There was no decrease in mortality for users of vitamin C alone (*American Journal of Clinical Nutrition,* August 1996).

VITAMIN E AND THE CARDIOVASCULAR SYSTEM

Q: It sounds like vitamin E was the key player in that study, and you did say that vitamin E's ability to protect the heart is gaining support. What's the story?

A: The claim that vitamin E protects the heart began in the 1940s when two Canadian physicians, brothers Evan and Wilfrid Shute, claimed that large doses of vitamin E were beneficial for treating heart disease and preventing heart attacks. The Shutes did not prove their claims to the satisfaction of the medical establishment, however.

Q: Were any studies ever done to test their theory?

A: Over the years, a number of studies looked at vitamin E and heart disease, with conflicting results as the following pairs of studies show.

- A 1987 World Health Organization (WHO) study found that people in countries where there is a high risk of

coronary heart disease—such as Scotland and Finland—
had low levels of vitamin E in their plasma, while
people in countries where there is a low risk of coronary heart disease—such as France and Italy—had high
plasma levels of vitamin E. In direct contradiction to
the WHO study, a 1988 Finnish study found that blood
levels of vitamin E were similar in men with and without coronary heart disease.

- Conflicting results were also found in two **case control studies** published in the journal *Lancet*. In the first study, published in 1991, researchers reported that blood levels of vitamin E were significantly lower in people with **angina** (chest pain caused by lack of oxygen to the heart) than in a comparable group of healthy people. In fact, the researchers reported that those with the lowest vitamin E levels were 2.7 times more likely to develop angina. But in the other study, reported in 1993, researchers compared tissue concentrations of vitamin E in people who had just had heart attacks with those of healthy individuals and found no difference.

Q: When did vitamin E's heart-protective effects begin to gain wider acceptance?

A: The turnaround came in 1993 when Harvard University researchers published two landmark studies that brought vitamin E into the public eye.

- The Nurses' Health Study followed the dietary habits and health status of 87,245 female nurses for eight years and found that those who had the highest intake of vitamin E were 36 percent less likely to develop heart disease than were those who had the lowest intake. The highest benefits were seen in women who took supplements; in fact, only those who took supplements for at least two years showed a benefit (*New England Journal of Medicine,* May 20, 1993).

- The Health Professionals Follow-up Study, similar in design to the Nurses' Health Study, followed 39,910 male health professionals for four years and found that those who took in the most vitamin E per day were approximately 40 percent less likely to develop heart disease than were those who didn't. Those who took in at least 100 I.U. of vitamin E per day for at least two years saw the most benefit (*New England Journal of Medicine,* May 20, 1993).

Q: That's pretty impressive. But why were these studies more important than those conflicting ones that preceded them?

A: These studies had weight primarily because of their size—thousands of people participated in them—and because of their length—they lasted for years.

Q: Have any other studies resulted in similar findings?

A: Yes. By early 1995, seven major studies had shown that high intake or blood levels of vitamin E lowered the risk of death from heart disease, while three studies that looked specifically at blood levels of vitamin E did not find a clear association (*Lancet,* January 21, 1995).

Q: It sounds like intake is the key here. Am I right?

A: Perhaps. The majority of studies that have looked at vitamin E intake have linked higher intakes—particularly from supplements—to a reduced risk of heart disease.

Q: So is it widely accepted that vitamin E supplements can reduce the risk of heart disease?

A: Not exactly. The picture is a little more complicated than that, thanks in large part to researchers at the University of Minnesota School of Public Health in Minneapolis.

Q: What did those researchers find?

A: The researchers conducted a seven-year study of 34,486 postmenopausal women similar in design to the Nurses' Health Study and the Health Professionals Follow-up Study. They surveyed the women on their dietary intakes and monitored their health for an extended period of time. They found that while those who took in the most vitamin E reduced their risk of dying from heart disease, the highest reduction in risk was in the 21,809 women who *did not* take supplements. In those women, the highest vitamin E intake corresponded to a 58 percent reduction in risk. After the researchers adjusted the figure to take into account other risk factors, these women still had a 52 percent risk reduction. There was little evidence that vitamin E supplements decreased risk (*New England Journal of Medicine,* May 2, 1996).

Q: That really seems to contradict those two Harvard studies. Did the researchers provide any explanation for the discrepancy?

A: Yes. While newspapers across the country ran headlines that vitamin E supplements don't appear to protect the heart, the researchers quietly noted that their study didn't specifically address high-dose supplementation or duration of supplement use.

"We had no information on the duration of supplement intake," the researchers wrote, adding that other studies found a benefit only in people who had been taking supplements for at least two years. "In addition," they wrote, "relatively few women in our cohort consumed high doses of supplemental vitamin E."

Q: Does that mean supplements might help reduce the risk of heart disease?

A: It's certainly possible, but experts will not know for certain until they conduct the most rigorous type of study—a **placebo-controlled study**. This type of study compares the effectiveness of a specific treatment to the effectiveness of a **placebo**, or inactive, treatment.

Q: I guess there's no clear answer to my question, but it certainly looks like vitamin E has some sort of heart-protective effect. Do experts have any idea exactly how vitamin E may protect the heart?

A: Yes. In fact, they have several pretty strong hypotheses. Among the most widely accepted is the theory that vitamin E prevents the oxidation of **low-density lipoprotein (LDL)**, the so-called bad **cholesterol**. Oxidized LDL has been linked to the development of **atherosclerosis**, a buildup of **plaque**, or fatty deposits, on artery walls that contributes to **coronary-artery disease** and stroke.

Q: Anything else?

A: Yes. Vitamin E may also help to prevent later stages of atherosclerosis by preventing white blood cells, known as **leukocytes**, from adhering to artery walls and by preventing the excessive formation of smooth muscle cells in damaged arteries. It may improve the function of the blood vessels themselves by protecting the **endothelium**, the cells that line the inner walls of arteries, from oxidative damage. And it may prevent blood clots by preventing **platelets**, small disk-shaped objects in the blood, from clumping together.

Vitamin E and Atherosclerosis

Q: That's quite an array of theories, and I'm not up enough on the mechanics of the heart and blood vessels to understand them all. Could we break things down and look at them one at a time?

A: Certainly. Let's start with the mechanics. Many of the theories on how vitamin E protects the heart originate from its role in atherosclerosis, a buildup of plaque on artery walls that can clog arteries and prevent oxygen-rich blood from flowing through. If the buildup is in arteries that bring blood to the heart, atherosclerosis can lead to angina or heart attack. If the buildup is in the **carotid arteries**, the arteries in the neck that bring blood to the brain, it can lead to stroke.

Q: How does this plaque build up?

A: The most widely held theory is that atherosclerosis begins when excess LDL circulating in the bloodstream begins to stick to artery walls, generally in areas where the endothelium has been damaged.

Q: How does the endothelium get damaged?

A: There are a number of ways. High blood pressure, toxins from cigarette smoke, and bacterial or viral infections can produce microscopic tears or rough spots. Areas where blood flow is turbulent are also susceptible to damage.

Q: Is that all that happens? The LDL just piles up on artery walls?

A: No. It appears to be much more complex than that. Once the LDL is there, many researchers believe, it squeezes through the spaces between the endothelial cells until it is inside the wall of the artery. There, it reacts with oxygen, creating potentially harmful free radicals. This process, known as lipid peroxidation, sets off a chain reaction that attracts more LDL cholesterol.

Q: Then what?

A: At this point, researchers believe, cells known as **macrophages** move in to "eat up" the oxidized LDL cholesterol. Once they become full, they turn into large, fluffy cells known as **foam cells**. These foam cells die, spilling their contents within the artery wall. This causes cracks in the artery wall that attract platelets, which secrete chemicals that attract smooth muscle cells. These cells proliferate and form scar tissue. Finally, calcium from the bloodstream may cover the whole mess with a hard shell.

Q: No wonder the arteries get blocked! But from that list of theories you spouted off, it sounds like vitamin E may be able to affect the process in several ways. Have any studies looked at whether or not vitamin E actually has an effect on atherosclerosis?

A: Yes. Several studies indicate that vitamin E may reduce the severity or slow the progression of atherosclerosis.

- Researchers at the University of Southern California School of Medicine, Los Angeles, in 1996 reported preliminary data from an ongoing study of heart disease risks in 56 men and women. In the first year of the study, the researchers found that study participants taking vitamin E supplements at doses of approximately 100 I.U. a day had less plaque buildup in their carotid arteries than would be expected based on their ages and other risk factors. Lisa Nicholson, R.D., one of the study researchers, told *Science News* (May 4, 1996) that the supplements appear to have reduced plaque buildup by an amount "equivalent to about 14 years of aging."

- In the Cholesterol Lowering Atherosclerosis Study (CLAS), researchers recruited 146 men who had had coronary-artery bypass graft surgery and assigned half to receive a cholesterol-lowering drug and half to receive a placebo. All of the men were instructed on how to eat an appropriate diet. During the course of the two-year study, researchers measured the thickness of the carotid artery walls in the men to see if atherosclerosis was progressing. They also looked at the men's self-reported use of supplements. The researchers found that men who took 100 I.U. of vitamin E or more were less likely to experience a thickening of their artery walls. This was most apparent in men who didn't take cholesterol-lowering drugs, leading researchers to believe that the effects of the drug therapy overpowered the effects of vitamin E supplements.

- A study reported in *Atherosclerosis* (January 1995) found that atherosclerotic lesions in coronary arteries were less severe in people with higher blood levels of vitamin E than in people with low blood levels of vitamin E.

- Researchers studied vitamin E's effects on 50 people with atherosclerosis in their carotid arteries by giving them either vitamin E or a placebo. When they measured the thickness of the plaque buildup at six and 12 months using an ultrasound scan, they found that atherosclerosis had regressed in seven of the 25 people given vitamin E and progressed in two. In contrast, none of the participants who received the placebo experienced regression, and 10 experienced progression (*Lipids,* December 1995).

Vitamin E and Cholesterol

Q: I'd like to know more about *how* vitamin E affects atherosclerosis. Didn't you say it may have some effect on cholesterol?

A: Yes. Vitamin E is thought to prevent or slow the oxidation of LDL cholesterol—the kind of cholesterol that sticks to artery walls.

Q: I can understand why experts think vitamin E might do that—it is, after all, an antioxidant—but is there any evidence that it actually does?

A: Yes. British researchers who compared the vitamin E content of atherosclerotic lesions with that of normal arterial walls found that the level of vitamin E was lower in the lesions, particularly those rich in foam cells. Because of this and because there was an accumulation of oxidized by-products in the lesions, they concluded that significant oxidation of LDL cholesterol occurs in the lesions only after vitamin E has been depleted (*Free Radical Research,* December 1995).

Q: That's all well and good, but have any studies found a direct effect?

A: Yes. Several studies indicate that vitamin E increases LDL's resistance to oxidation—in other words, it makes LDL less susceptible to oxidation.

Q: How do researchers measure this susceptibility?

A: By looking at the rate of oxidation and the amount of time it takes for oxidation to occur.

Q: What exactly have the researchers found?

A: Here's a sampling.

- Researchers investigating the minimal dose of vitamin E necessary to protect LDL from oxidation in test tubes gave 20 healthy volunteers 25, 50, 100, 200, 400 and 800 I.U. of vitamin E daily. An analysis of their blood revealed that the rate of oxidation was significantly decreased at doses of 400 and 800 I.U. (*Arteriosclerosis, Thrombosis and Vascular Biology,* March 1995).

- Australian researchers added vitamin E to LDL in test tubes and induced oxidation. They found that the vitamin generated a nearly threefold increase in lag time (the time it takes for oxidation to occur). It also reduced the amount of LDL that accumulated in macrophages (*Atherosclerosis,* September 1994).

- In a study reported in the December 1993 *Circulation,* people given 800 I.U. of vitamin E, 1,000 milligrams of vitamin C and 30 milligrams of beta carotene per day experienced a 40 percent decrease in the oxidation rate of their blood fats, or lipids. Those who received 800 I.U. of vitamin E alone experienced similar results.

- In a 12-week study, 45 people with cardiovascular disease were given either a placebo or one of two combinations of antioxidant supplements: a dose containing 400 I.U. of vitamin E, 500 milligrams of vitamin C and 12 milligrams of beta carotene; or a high dose containing 800 I.U. of vitamin E, 1,000 milligrams of vitamin C and 24 milligrams of beta carotene. The researchers then examined the subjects' blood to see if the supplements had any effect on LDL oxidation. They found that the amount of time it took until oxidation occurred increased significantly in the people who received the high dose of supplements (*Journal of the American College of Cardiology,* August 1997).

- Researchers who conducted test-tube studies of the blood of Scottish men found that the red blood cells of those who smoked were more susceptible to lipid peroxidation than were the red blood cells of those who didn't smoke. When both the smokers' and nonsmokers' diets were supplemented with 70, 140, 560 and 1,050 milligrams of vitamin E for 20 weeks, the level of vitamin E in their red blood cells increased. In the smokers, each dose was associated with a significant decrease in the susceptibility of their blood cells to oxidation. The nonsmokers' blood cells also experienced decreased susceptibility, except at the highest dose. At that dose, the nonsmokers' blood cells experienced an increase in susceptibility to oxidation (*American Journal of Clinical Nutrition,* February 1997).

Q: **Those studies sound pretty promising, but that last one has me a little confused. How could vitamin E trigger an increase in susceptibility to oxidation?**

A: Several studies indicate that under certain circumstances, vitamin E can act as a **pro-oxidant**, rather than an antioxidant. A pro-oxidant is a substance that encourages or speeds up oxidation.

Q: How can vitamin E act as a pro-oxidant?

A: As you may recall from chapter 1, oxidation occurs when unstable molecules or atoms known as free radicals steal electrons from other molecules or atoms. As an antioxidant, vitamin E donates electrons to these free radicals, thus stopping their thieving behavior. In the process, vitamin E itself becomes unbalanced. Generally, this simply renders it inactive. But in certain situations, this lack of balance causes it to promote oxidation.

Q: What are those certain situations?

A: The researchers of the Scottish study believe that vitamin E may promote oxidation when the amount of vitamin E in red blood cells increases more than 200 percent and there is not a corresponding increase of vitamin C. (There is evidence that vitamin C regenerates oxidized vitamin E, returning it to its potent antioxidant state.) Other studies suggest that vitamin E becomes pro-oxidant when an unstable, oxidized form of vitamin E, the **alpha-tocopheroxyl radical**, is isolated in an individual LDL particle without an antioxidant to neutralize it (*Journal of Biological Chemistry*, March 17, 1995).

Q: Does this occur often?

A: Apparently not. A study reported in *FEBS Letters* (March 6, 1995) found that vitamin E is converted to alpha-tocopheroxyl when it reacts with either copper or a peroxyl radical (a specific free radical). Because this only occurs in the presence of copper and low levels of lipid hydroperoxides, the researchers said, the pro-oxidant quality of vitamin E is not a significant factor for most people. In most cases, vitamin E stops or slows down—rather than speeds up—the oxidation of LDL cholesterol.

Q: That's good. Does vitamin E have any other effect on cholesterol? I seem to recall reading somewhere that it might affect cholesterol levels.

A: There have been claims that vitamin E can lower LDL cholesterol levels and increase the amount of **high-density lipoprotein (HDL)**, the type of cholesterol that helps transport excess cholesterol out of the body, but the evidence is inconclusive. While one study found that 500 I.U. of vitamin E can raise HDL cholesterol by about 14 percent, another study failed to produce similar results. And while a study from the Harvard Medical School did find that vitamin E supplements of 800 I.U. per day produce a slight decrease in LDL levels, the researchers concluded that vitamin E does not affect blood levels of lipids (such as cholesterol) in normal adults.

Vitamin E and White Blood Cells

Q: How else is vitamin E thought to protect against atherosclerosis?

A: Vitamin E may help prevent white blood cells from adhering to artery walls. Studies show that the white blood cells of people who have been given vitamin E do not stick to artery walls as much as the white blood cells of people who have not been given vitamin E do, according to an article on the role of antioxidants in atherosclerotic heart disease (*New England Journal of Medicine,* August 7, 1997).

Vitamin E and Smooth Muscle Cells

Q: Does vitamin E have any other effects on plaque buildup?

A: It appears to. As we mentioned earlier, vitamin E prevents the excessive proliferation of smooth muscle cells that contributes to plaque buildup.

Q: Is this another of vitamin E's antioxidant functions?

A: No. In this instance, vitamin E appears to work by decreasing the activity of **protein kinase C**, an enzyme that stimulates the production of smooth muscle cells.

Swiss researchers who studied the effects of vitamin E on protein kinase C activity in the smooth muscle cells of rats found that vitamin E prevents the activation of protein kinase C (*Proceedings of the National Academy of Sciences,* December 19, 1995).

Vitamin E and Blood Vessels

Q: We've discussed the substances that stick to artery walls. Does vitamin E have any direct effect on the arteries themselves?

A: Vitamin E appears to protect the endothelium—the cells that line artery walls—from damage and dysfunction. Atherosclerosis is known to damage these cells, causing them to function improperly. For example, endothelial cells that have been damaged by atherosclerosis do not dilate properly, which can impede blood flow.

Q: What happens to these damaged cells when vitamin E is present?

A: According to one animal study, vitamin E may help the cells respond to **vasodilators**, vessel-dilating drugs that are often given to people with coronary-artery disease to prevent heart attack. In the study, Swedish researchers gave rabbits cholesterol in an effort to induce endothelial dysfunction; they then gave some of the rabbits vitamin E. When they administered a vessel-dilating drug to the rabbits, the drug had little effect on the rabbits that were not given vitamin E, but it worked on those that were given vitamin E. The researchers concluded that vitamin E may help prevent further deterioration of endothelial function and may help reverse the effects of high cholesterol levels, which contribute to atherosclerosis (*Atherosclerosis,* November 1994).

Q: Have any human studies found that vitamin E improves the function of blood vessels?

A: Yes. In a study that was published, ironically, the day before Thanksgiving, researchers from the University of Maryland School of Medicine reported that treatment with vitamins E and C can prevent endothelial dysfunction caused by a high-fat meal (*Journal of the American Medical Association,* November 26, 1997).

The researchers gave 20 healthy people with normal cholesterol levels a high-fat breakfast or a low-fat breakfast, with or without 800 I.U. of vitamin E and 1,000 milligrams of vitamin C. They then used ultrasound to measure the dilation in the participants' brachial arteries (the major arteries in the arms) for six hours following the meal. They found that the high-fat meal reduced arterial dilation for up to four hours— but not when it was given with the vitamins.

Q: I assume that's good, but I'm not sure why. Why did the high-fat meal affect the blood vessels, and how did the vitamins prevent this effect?

A: The researchers theorize that the high-fat diet may have caused **triglycerides**, fatty compounds, to accumulate, triggering an oxidative reaction that impaired the endothelial cells' ability to function correctly. They concluded that vitamin E and vitamin C, both antioxidants, may have prevented the dysfunction by blocking the oxidative reaction.

Vitamin E and the Blood

Q: OK. So vitamin E appears to help blood vessels function correctly. Didn't you also say that it may help prevent blood clots?

A: Yes, we did. Studies have shown that vitamin E decreases platelets' tendency to stick together and to stick to other substances. This tendency is an important part of blood clotting, which helps prevent blood loss. But it can also contribute to atherosclerosis as well as heart attack and stroke.

Q: How exactly does vitamin E affect platelets?

A: Test-tube studies show that vitamin E affects platelet function in a variety of very technical ways: To put it simply, the vitamin plays a role in the creation, activity, metabolism and amount of a number of biochemical substances crucial for platelet function; and either vitamin E or one of its derivatives may also play a direct role in stopping platelets from clumping together.

Q: What do you mean, "one of its derivatives"?

A: When vitamin E is involved in an oxidative reaction, it donates electrons to free radicals, thus changing its composition. One of the molecules that it can become, **vitamin E quinone**, appears to be a potent anticoagulant. In other words, it appears to prevent or delay blood clotting.

Q: How does it do this?

A: According to one theory, vitamin E quinone inhibits an enzyme that modifies a variety of proteins in order for clots to form. Some researchers believe it does this by binding to the site on the enzyme where vitamin K—which is crucial in blood clotting—usually attaches. Whatever the mechanism, however, vitamin E and, perhaps, its derivative appear to stop platelets from clumping together, or aggregating, and from sticking to a variety of substances.

Q: How do we know this?

A: Studies show that decreased blood levels of vitamin E are associated with increased clumping of platelets—an increase that is reversed when blood levels of vitamin E increase. Other studies have found that high levels of vitamin E reduce platelets' tendency to stick to a variety of adhesive proteins.

Q: Have any studies looked directly at the effects vitamin E supplements have on platelet function?

A: Yes. Here are two.

- A study reported in *Atherosclerosis* (January 1997) looked at the effects that daily supplementation with 300 milligrams of vitamin E, 250 milligrams of vitamin C and 15 milligrams of beta carotene for eight weeks had on the platelet function of 40 healthy adults. The researchers found that supplementation with vitamin E increased both plasma and platelet levels of vitamin E. The researchers also found that their ability to cause platelets to clump together was decreased after the study participants took vitamin E. They concluded that supplementation with antioxidants—particularly vitamin E—might help prevent blood clots and atherosclerosis in people who have low dietary intakes of vitamin E and could benefit older people and people with diabetes, whose platelets have a greater tendency to clump together.

- Finnish researchers who assigned 80 men with low blood levels of antioxidants to receive either a placebo or 300 milligrams of vitamin E, 600 milligrams of vitamin C, 27 milligrams of beta carotene and 75 micrograms of selenium for five months found that the men who took the supplements had a 24 percent decrease in their platelets' tendency to clump together as well as significant decreases in biochemicals that regulate platelet function and a 20 percent decrease in blood levels of a by-product of lipid peroxidation (*American Journal of Clinical Nutrition,* May 1991).

Vitamin E and Blood Flow

Q: It seems like there's more to vitamin E's heart-protective role than simply preventing or slowing the progression of atherosclerosis. Am I right?

A: Yes. Vitamin E's effect on platelets, as we said, may be instrumental in reducing the development of blood clots that can lead to heart attack and stroke. And the vitamin's ability to protect artery walls may have an impact on blood flow. Indeed, vitamin E has been shown in several studies to reduce blood clots and improve circulation and has been used to treat **thrombophlebitis** and **intermittent claudication**.

Q: What is thrombophlebitis?

A: Thrombophlebitis is the swelling of a vein along with the formation of a clot. Thrombophlebitis is often caused by an increased clotting ability in blood, which is why vitamin E has been used to treat it.

Q: And intermittent claudication? What is that?

A: Intermittent claudication is a cramping pain in the calves and legs caused by poor circulation. In one study, supplementation with doses of 300 to 800 I.U. per day for at least three months resulted in improvement: Study participants who took the supplements saw improved blood flow in their leg arteries, were able to walk without pain and experienced fewer amputations than participants who took other substances or a placebo.

Q: Didn't you say earlier that vitamin E may also have an effect on angina?

A: Claims that vitamin E can alleviate the pain of angina (chest pain caused by lack of oxygen to the heart, often as a result of atherosclerosis or arterial contractions) have been made since the 1940s, but the evidence that vitamin E can relieve the pain of angina remains inconclusive.

Studies conducted in the 1970s indicate that vitamin E

cannot relieve angina symptoms, but more recent studies have found a link between low blood levels of vitamin E and angina.

- As we mentioned earlier, a 1991 study found that the study participants with the lowest blood levels of vitamin E were 2.7 times more likely to develop angina than were those with the highest blood levels.

- A study reported in the March 6, 1996, *Journal of the American Medical Association* found that male smokers who took 50 milligrams of vitamin E for four years were 9 percent less likely to develop angina than were their counterparts who took a placebo.

- Japanese researchers who studied men and women with active angina, inactive angina and no coronary-artery disease found that those with active angina had lower blood levels of vitamin E than did those who were pain-free or disease-free. Those who were experiencing pain were given a drug used to treat angina. Vitamin E levels rose in those who were helped by the drug. When those who still experienced pain with the medication were given 300 I.U. of vitamin E per day for two weeks, their vitamin E levels rose and the frequency of their angina attacks was reduced (*Circulation,* July 1, 1996).

Vitamin E and Heart Disease

Q: We started out discussing whether or not vitamin E reduces the risk of heart disease, but now we seem to be talking about its effects on heart disease—after all, angina is a symptom of heart disease. Does vitamin E have any benefit for people with heart disease?

A: It appears so. As we've seen, vitamin E may slow the progression of atherosclerosis, which can lessen the severity of coronary-artery disease and reduce the risk of angina. It may also improve blood flow and prevent the development of blood clots, which can lead to heart attacks.

Q: Has anyone looked at whether vitamin E is effective in preventing heart attacks or reducing the complications of heart disease?

A: Yes. The Cambridge Heart Antioxidant Study compared the effectiveness of vitamin E in doses of 400 or 800 I.U. with the effectiveness of a placebo in 2,002 men and women with coronary-artery disease. Those who took vitamin E for 18 months were 47 percent less likely to die of heart-related problems or to have a nonfatal heart attack than were those who took the placebo. In fact, they were 77 percent less likely to have a nonfatal heart attack (*Lancet,* March 23, 1996).

A recent analysis of data from a widely publicized 1994 study that linked beta carotene to lung cancer also indicated that vitamin E supplements might reduce the risk of nonfatal heart attack, but the analysis found no connection between vitamin E supplements and fatal heart attacks or other fatal coronary events. The analysis, published in the June 14, 1997, *Lancet,* looked at the frequency of coronary events in 1,862 Finnish men who had previously had heart attacks and found that 50-milligram supplements of vitamin E, either alone or with beta carotene, did not reduce the risk of death from heart-related problems. They did, however, reduce the risk of nonfatal heart attack by 38 percent. Earlier results from this study, which evaluated the supplements' effect on 29,133 Finnish smokers regardless of their heart history, found that the vitamin E supplements conferred only a 5 percent reduction in coronary mortality—a reduction the researchers considered nonsignificant.

Q: Have any experts theorized why the results of this Finnish study are so much less promising than those of the British study or those large Harvard studies?

A: Yes. In an article published in the December 1995 supplement of the *American Journal of Clinical Nutrition,* Meir J. Stampfer and Eric B. Rimm, the lead researchers, respectively, of the Nurses' Health and Health Professionals Follow-up studies, state that while some people have interpreted the Finnish findings as disproving the theory that vitamin E protects against coronary heart disease, "the results are entirely consistent" with those observed in the two Harvard studies. In those studies, they noted, "the intake of low doses of vitamin E, in the range used in the Finnish trial, also was not associated with any material decrease in the risk of heart disease.... Hence, the Finnish trial did not provide an adequate test of the hypothesis because of the low dose of vitamin E that was used." The researchers go on to note that both Harvard studies and the Finnish study "suggest that the major effect, if any, is mainly found with an intake greater than or equal to 100 I.U. per day," which, they say, could explain the inconsistent results found in studies that look at blood levels of vitamin E.

"Because vitamin E has little toxicity, this research represents a promising approach to prevention of coronary heart disease. If the true magnitude of such an effect is similar to that observed in the Health Professionals Follow-up Study and the Nurses' Health Study, then vitamin E supplementation could have a major effect on the incidence of coronary heart disease."

—Meir J. Stampfer and Eric B. Rimm
American Journal of Clinical Nutrition
December 1995 supplement

Vitamin E and Stroke

Q: It sounds like it's possible that vitamin E may reduce the risk of heart attack. Does it have any effect on stroke risk?

A: Yes. Many of the risk factors for heart attack—atherosclerosis, high cholesterol and an increased tendency to form blood clots, for example—are also risk factors for stroke—as is heart disease itself. Consequently, any effect vitamin E has on these risk factors is likely to translate into an effect on stroke risk.

Q: Is the effect a beneficial one?

A: For the most part, yes. We've already discussed several studies that found that vitamin E slowed the progression of atherosclerosis in the carotid arteries. Blockage of these arteries, which supply blood to the brain, is a major cause of **ischemic stroke**, the most common kind of stroke. And a number of studies indicate that adequate vitamin E intake reduces the risk of or death rate from ischemic stroke.

Q: What kind of reductions do these studies show?

A: Here are a few examples.

- The Chinese Cancer Prevention Trial, which analyzed the effects of antioxidant supplements in rural Chinese men and women, found that study participants given 30 milligrams of vitamin E, along with 15 milligrams of beta carotene and 50 micrograms of selenium, were 10 percent less likely to die from stroke during the study period than were those who did not receive the supplements (*American Journal of Clinical Nutrition,* December 1995).

- In a Japanese study, 2,271 stroke survivors were given either conventional treatment or 600 milligrams of dl-alpha-tocopherol nicotinate, a molecule that is part vitamin E and part nicotinic acid (a form of the vitamin niacin) for three years. Those who received the supplements had a lower overall incidence of fatal and nonfatal stroke than did those who received the placebo. They also had lower a lower incidence of heart disease and death from any cause.

- Researchers from the East Carolina University School of Medicine gave 100 people who experienced transient ischemic attacks (temporary strokelike events) or minor strokes either aspirin alone or aspirin plus 400 I.U. of vitamin E for two years in an effort to protect against future **cerebrovascular** problems. Those who received the vitamin in combination with aspirin were less likely to have a stroke than were those who received the aspirin alone. (Aspirin is known to reduce stroke risk and is a common treatment for preventing stroke.) The researchers theorized that the reduction in risk was caused by the reduction in platelets adhering to vessel walls (*American Journal of Clinical Nutrition,* December 1995 supplement).

Q: That sounds promising. Why did you use the words "for the most part" when you said vitamin E has a beneficial effect on stroke?

A: Because there is some evidence that vitamin E can increase the risk of **hemorrhagic stroke**, the type of stroke caused by the rupture or leakage of blood vessels in or on the brain.

Q: What's the evidence?

A: The 1994 Finnish study we discussed earlier found an increase in the death rate from hemorrhagic stroke in men who took vitamin E supplements, a finding researchers attributed to vitamin E's effects on platelets.

Q: I hadn't thought of that. I guess it's not always good to improve blood flow, is it?

A: Not always. Because vitamin E does function as an anticoagulant, people who are taking anticoagulant drugs, people with vitamin K deficiencies (as you may recall, vitamin K is crucial for blood clotting, and vitamin E may compete with it) and people whose blood does not clot normally should not take vitamin E supplements unless they're under a doctor's care.

Q: Even with that cautionary note in mind, it seems like vitamin E may be of real benefit to the cardiovascular system. Could you help me put this all in perspective by summarizing exactly how vitamin E is thought to benefit the heart and blood vessels?

A: Certainly. Studies indicate that vitamin E may protect the heart and blood vessels by doing the following:

- protecting LDL cholesterol from oxidizing
- preventing white blood cells from sticking to artery walls
- maintaining or improving the function of blood vessels
- preventing the excessive proliferation of smooth muscle cells
- preventing platelets from clumping together and adhering to other substances

VITAMIN E AND THE IMMUNE SYSTEM

Q: You've said that vitamin E plays a role in improving immune response. Is that how it protects against other diseases?

A: It's one way, yes. The immune system is our body's system of defense against bacteria, viruses and other harmful invaders that cause disease—including infections and cancer.

Q: What parts of the body play a role in the immune system?

A: The major components of the immune system include the bone marrow and the **thymus** gland, which manufacture and process white blood cells; the tissues, vessels, organs and nodes of the lymphatic system, which filters and conveys a fluid known as lymph and produces various types of white blood cells; and the white blood cells themselves. These cells, known as leukocytes, are present throughout the body in blood and lymph and play an important role in fending off foreign substances.

Q: What do these blood cells do?

A: That depends on the type of cell. There are several different kinds of leukocytes, and each plays a different role in the immune response.

B lymphocytes, or B cells, are responsible for a type of immune response known as **humoral immunity**. They identify potentially harmful foreign substances, known as **antigens**, and attempt to render them harmless. They do this by producing **antibodies**, which attach to the antigens and neutralize them much in the way antioxidants neutralize free radicals.

T lymphocytes, or T cells, initiate, direct and terminate a type of immune response known as **cell-mediated immunity**. They stimulate B cells to produce antibodies and to attack and kill invaders within specific cells. T cells also destroy invaders directly and produce chemicals called **lymphokines**, which stimulate **phagocytes** to attack and kill invaders.

Phagocytes are cells that engulf, or ingest, bacteria, viruses, cell fragments and abnormal cells such as those that lead to cancer. Macrophages, which eat up oxidized LDL cholesterol and contribute to atherosclerosis, are a type of phagocyte.

Q: That sounds like quite an army. Are any other troops involved?

A: Yes. Other chemicals are also crucial to the function of the immune system. These chemicals, known as **mediators**, are released from cells when foreign substances meet up with antibodies or T cells. Their release can trigger a variety of bodily reactions, including inflammation, changes in blood pressure and dilation or contraction of blood vessels.

Vitamin E and Immune Response

Q: How does vitamin E come into play in all this?

A: Studies show that vitamin E is essential for the normal function of the immune system: Deficiencies of vitamin E are associated with decreased immune response.

Q: Before we go any further, can you explain what you mean by "immune response"?

A: Immune response is the body's defense against invading antigens and cancer. In other words, immune response is the way the immune system functions. We outlined the two types of immune response—humoral and cell-mediated immunity—in our discussion of the roles played by the various parts of the immune system.

Q: OK. Now, what exactly happens to the immune response when people are deficient in vitamin E?

A: In some people with vitamin E deficiency, notably preterm infants, phagocytes don't function correctly, the immune system's ability to use oxidation to fight against foreign invaders and kill bacteria is depressed, and there is a decrease in the immune system cells' movement toward various stimuli, including foreign invaders (*Lancet,* January 21, 1995).

Q: Do scientists have any idea why this happens?

A: Yes. Without adequate vitamin E, the immune system is not sufficiently protected against oxidative damage; this causes defects in the membrane stability of immune system cells and results in an increase in the production of **prostaglandin E_2** and other biochemicals that suppress the activity of immune system.

> *"Data from clinical trials show that vitamin E supplementation or intakes above the RDA can increase the immune response, and this in turn may provide protection against cancer and infectious diseases."*
>
> —Mohsen Meydani, Ph.D.
> *Lancet,* January 21, 1995

Q: Wait a minute. What is prostaglandin E_2, and how does it suppress the immune system?

A: Prostaglandin E_2 is one of several prostaglandins—strong hormonelike fatty acids in the body. It suppresses the production of **interleukin-1** and **interleukin-2**, beneficial immune system mediators that activate and cause the proliferation of T and B lymphocytes. Prostaglandin E_2 also suppresses the proliferation of the lymphocytes themselves.

Q: You said that production of prostaglandin E_2 increases when there's a vitamin E deficiency. Does vitamin E have any direct effect on its production?

A: Yes. Vitamin E has been shown in test-tube studies to reduce the production of prostaglandin E_2 in immune cells, which, in turn, increases the production of interleukins and the proliferation of lymphocytes, thus improving immune response.

Q: Does vitamin E affect any other players in immune response?

A: Yes. Vitamin E has been shown to increase blood levels of immunoglobulin G (an antibody produced in response to bacteria, fungi and viruses) in healthy elderly women. Supplemental vitamin E has also been shown to aid in the production of some mediators, including interleukin-1. Researchers found that people who received 400 milligrams of vitamin E and 1,000 milligrams of vitamin C for 28 days had an increased production of interleukin-1 and an anticancer mediator known as tumor necrosis factor alpha (*American Journal of Clinical Nutrition,* December 1996).

Q: Does any of this translate into improved immune response?

A: Yes. Vitamin E has been shown to improve immune response—particularly cell-mediated immunity—in both animals and people.

Q: Let's start with the animals. What effects does vitamin E have on their immune response?

A: Here's what some recent studies have shown:

- Mice with AIDS were infected with a virus, then fed either a regular diet or a diet high in vitamin E for 10 weeks. Those fed the regular diet had larger spleens and a greater decrease in immune cell activity than those given the vitamin E-rich diet. And those given vitamin E had an increased production of beneficial immune system mediators and a better ratio of T cells. The researchers said their findings suggest that vitamin E normalizes the decrease of immune function that follows the development of AIDS in mice (*Nutrition Research*, October 1996).

- Japanese researchers fed rats a regular diet or a diet high in vitamin E for one year, then measured the functioning of their immune systems. They found that measures of immune system function were lower in older rats fed the regular diet than in younger rats fed the regular diet. But the measures were similar in old and young rats fed the diet high in vitamin E. As a result of the specific findings, the researchers theorize that vitamin E may be able to improve the decreased cellular immune function caused by aging (*Journal of Nutritional Science and Vitaminology*, February 1997).

- In a study of mice exposed to the influenza virus, older mice fed high doses of vitamin E in the two months prior to exposure had lower levels of the virus in their lungs than older mice given smaller amounts of vitamin E. The benefit occurred only in older mice, not in younger mice, leading Tufts University researchers to speculate that since older people have less resistance to the flu than younger people, they may benefit from vitamin E supplementation.

Q: That sounds promising. Have any of the human studies found similar benefits?

A: Yes. In recent years, a number of studies have indicated that vitamin E improves the immunity of elderly people, giving rise to claims that vitamin E can actually fight aging.

Q: What exactly have these studies shown?

A: Several studies have shown improved immune function in older people who have taken multivitamin supplements that include vitamin E.

- One study of healthy older people used delayed hypersensitivity skin tests to measure immune function. In these tests, the people were injected with small amounts of different antigens, substances that could cause infection or disease. When the immune system is functioning well, it produces antibodies to protect the body from the antigens and the infections or diseases they cause. The production of these antibodies produces a visible skin reaction, which indicates that the immune system is functioning well. In this study, reported in the September 1994 *American Journal of Clinical Nutrition,* the number of reactions to this test increased in healthy older people who took a standard multivitamin supplement—including 20 milligrams of vitamin E—once a day for a year.

- In a 1992 Canadian study, healthy older people who supplemented their diets with a multivitamin supplement that contained 44 milligrams of vitamin E saw a decrease in the number of days they were sick and the amount of antibiotics they used in addition to an increase in antibody response to the flu vaccine.

Q: Have any studies shown a benefit from vitamin E alone, rather than vitamin E in a multivitamin supplement?

A: Yes. Researchers at the U.S. Department of Agriculture's Human Research Center on Aging at Tufts University in Boston have conducted several studies on vitamin E alone.

- In a landmark study of vitamin E's effect on immune response in healthy elderly people, Tufts researchers found that daily doses of 800 I.U. enhanced the function of T cells.

- In another important study, 88 seniors were given either a placebo or 60, 200 or 800 milligrams of vitamin E per day. Immune response increased no matter what the dose, but the 200 milligram dose produced the best results. After four months, those who received 200 milligrams showed a 65 percent increase in responses to delayed hypersensitivity skin tests. They also showed a sixfold increase in antibodies to hepatitis B after they were given a hepatitis B vaccine and a signficant increase in antibodies to tetanus. The researchers speculated that vitamin E enhanced T-cell function in healthy older people and noted that "recommendations to increase the intake of vitamin E for the elderly should be considered" (*Journal of the American Medical Association,* May 7, 1997).

Q: Why have all these vitamin E studies focused on the elderly?

A: Primarily because the elderly are more susceptible to infectious diseases and, so, may see more benefit from improved immune response.

"Many studies have shown that with aging, there is a dysregulation in parts of the immune system, which contributes to an increase in infectious diseases, an increase in tumors and to **autoimmune diseases** like arthritis," said Simin Nikbin Meydani, D.V.N., Ph.D., who headed the most recent Tufts study. "It is a big problem for the elderly. Infectious diseases such as pneumonia and influenza are among the leading causes of death in the elderly. What we've been trying to do is see if there are any dietary factors that can reverse the decline in the immune system with aging."

Vitamin E and Cancer

Q: The head researcher mentioned tumors. Does vitamin E's role in immune response relate directly to cancer prevention?

A: Yes. Remember: In addition to destroying bacteria and viruses, the immune system targets abnormal cells such as those that lead to cancer.

Q: I forgot about that. What exactly is the link between vitamin E and cancer?

A: While the evidence supporting vitamin E's protective effects against cancer is not as great as the evidence supporting its protective effects against heart disease, several links have been found. For instance, people with cancer often have lower blood levels of vitamin E than people without cancer. And some studies indicate that people who take in the most vitamin E—either from food or supplements—have less cancer risk than people who take in the least.

Vitamin E and Cancer Risk

Q: I'd like to know more about the studies that look at the links between vitamin E and cancer. Which cancers have researchers looked at, and what were the results?

A: Researchers have examined vitamin E's effect on lung, breast, colon and rectal cancer, with varying results. Studies have also noted connections between the vitamin and oral, stomach and prostate cancer.

Q: I'd like to look at the relationship between vitamin E and each of these cancers more closely, starting with lung cancer. Wasn't there a big study a few years back about vitamin E and lung cancer?

A: Yes. A highly publicized study looked at whether vitamin E—either alone or with beta carotene—could offer protection against lung cancer in men who smoke. The results of the study were disappointing. In fact, this is the Finnish study we discussed earlier. The Alpha-Tocopherol, Beta Carotene Cancer Prevention Study (ATBC), published in the April 14, 1994, *New England Journal of Medicine,* made headlines because the researchers found that the men who received beta carotene supplements had a *higher* incidence of lung cancer than did those who did not.

Q: Did vitamin E also increase lung cancer incidence?

A: No. But the researchers found no significant reduction in risk in the men who took vitamin E, which, you may recall, was given in doses of 50 milligrams per day.

Q: You did mention that before, and, actually, it confused me. I thought vitamin E was measured in international units. Why did the researchers in this study measure it in milligrams?

A: As you may recall from chapter 1, vitamin E comes in a variety of forms with varying potencies. To compare the various forms with one another, experts have used an arbitrary unit of measurement known as the international unit, which is also used to measure the various forms of vitamin A. More recently, another arbitrary unit—the tocopherol equivalent—has been used. This measure, which is specific to vitamin E, is generally provided in milligrams and is the form in which the Recommended Dietary Allowances (RDAs) appear. Thus, researchers have the option of measuring vitamin E in international units or in milligrams of tocopherol equivalents. The latter form is often simply referred to as milligrams.

Q: Thanks. Getting back to that 50-milligram per day dose, isn't that a rather small dose—at least compared with the doses used in other studies?

A: It is. In fact, the authors of the editorial that accompanied the study noted that the study should not be seen as proving vitamin E ineffective because the dose of vitamin E was small—smaller than the doses that have been shown in other studies to benefit the cardiovascular system. The editorial writers also pointed out that the vitamin was given in a synthetic form that is not readily absorbed and used by the body. As a result, blood levels of vitamin E increased by only about one-third in the study participants who received vitamin E supplements. In contrast, they noted, "a standard capsule of a vitamin E supplement contains a few hundred milligrams, and one or two capsules per day can double the blood level."

Q: That study doesn't seem to be very conclusive. Has there been any other research?

A: Yes. In fact, researchers recently reevaluated the data from the ATBC study to see if vitamin E offered benefits to any subgroups of study participants. Once again, they found no overall protective effect, but they did find that there was a lower incidence of lung cancer in people who had higher blood levels or intake of vitamin E at the beginning of the study. They also found that while there was no overall change in lung cancer incidence among those who took vitamin E, the occurrence of lung cancer was slightly lower when compared with that of men who didn't get vitamin E in the later years of the follow-up (*Journal of the National Cancer Institute,* November 6, 1996).

Q: That's all well and good, but we're still talking about the same study. Have there been any other studies?

A: Yes. Here are some of their findings.

- In one study, researchers compared the diets, smoking history and other risk factors of people with lung cancer with those of people without lung cancer and found that those who used vitamin E supplements had a 45 percent reduced risk of lung cancer (*Journal of the National Cancer Institute,* January 5, 1994).

- Researchers who looked at the relationship between dietary intake of vitamins E, C and A and lung cancer in some 10,000 men and women who answered a national health survey found that those with the highest dietary intake of all three vitamins were 68 percent less likely to develop lung cancer during the 19-year follow-up period than were those with the lowest intake. Smokers with the highest dietary intake of vitamin E were 64 percent less likely to develop lung cancer than were smokers with the lowest intake (*American Journal of Epidemiology,* August 1, 1997).

Q: What about the link between vitamin E and breast cancer?

A: Several studies have found a link between vitamin E levels and breast cancer.

- Turkish researchers who compared the blood levels of vitamin E in 100 women with breast cancer with those of 70 women without breast cancer found that the levels were significantly lower in the women with cancer (*Journal of Clinical Pharmacy and Therapeutics,* June 1995).

- A study reported in the *International Journal of Cancer* (July 17, 1996) looked at the levels of vitamin E in the breast tissue of women with and without breast cancer and found that the levels were significantly lower in the women with breast cancer.

Q: Have any studies looked specifically at vitamin E and breast cancer risk?

A: Yes, with mixed results.

- Researchers from the State University of New York at Buffalo reported in the September 1995 *Cancer Causes and Control* that women with a family history of breast cancer seemed to obtain some protection by taking in vitamin E. Those whose diets included the most vitamin E were 80 percent less likely to develop breast cancer than were those whose diets included the least. In women without a family of breast cancer, those with the highest vitamin E intake were 40 percent less likely to develop breast cancer than were those with the lowest intake. In this study, the highest intake was 10.4 I.U. or more—slightly under the RDA.

- In a study that compared the vitamin E intake of 297 women with breast cancer with that of 311 women without breast cancer, women whose diets were highest in vitamin E were 45 percent less likely to develop cancer than were those whose diets were lowest in vitamin E. But the researchers found no association between breast cancer risk and vitamin E intake from supplements (*Journal of the National Cancer Institute,* March 20, 1996).

- In studies conducted in two Chinese cities, researchers compared the diets of women with breast cancer with those of women without breast cancer and found no link between breast cancer and vitamin E intake (*British Journal of Cancer,* June 1995).

Q: What about colon and rectal cancer?

A: Here, too, study results are mixed.

- In the Finnish ATBC study, the men who took vitamin E supplements were 16 percent less likely to develop colorectal cancer than were those who did not.

- Researchers compared the diets of 1,326 Italians with colon or rectal cancer with those of 2,024 healthy individuals and found that those who took in the highest amount of vitamin E were 40 percent less likely to develop cancer than were those who took in the least amount.

- In a study that examined the relationship between diet and the risk of colorectal **polyps** (small growths that can lead to cancer), researchers compared the diets of 236 people with colorectal polyps or colorectal cancer with those of 409 healthy individuals and found that in men, those who took the most vitamin E were 65 percent less likely to develop polyps than were those who took in the least (*American Journal of Epidemiology*, December 1, 1996).

- Researchers randomly assigned 864 people with a history of colorectal polyps to receive one of four treatments: 400 milligrams of vitamin E and 1,000 milligrams of vitamin C; 25 milligrams of beta carotene; all three vitamins; or a placebo. They then performed exams to see how many study participants formed new polyps. They found that those who took the combination of vitamin E and vitamin C formed slightly more polyps than did those in the other groups (*New England Journal of Medicine*, July 21, 1994).

Q: Didn't you say researchers have also found a link between vitamin E and oral cancer?

A: Yes. In several epidemiologic studies, low intakes of vitamin E, **carotenoids** or both are associated with a higher risk of cancer of the oral cavity. And at least one study indicates that vitamin E and beta carotene can cause patchy lesions called leukoplakia to regress. These lesions may progress to cancer in some people (*American Journal of Clinical Nutrition*, December 1995 supplement).

Q: What about stomach and prostate cancers?

A: In the Chinese Cancer Prevention Study, 29,000 adults were randomly assigned to receive a placebo or supplements of vitamin E, beta carotene and selenium for approximately five years. Those who took the supplements were 21 percent less likely to die of stomach cancer and 9 percent less likely to die of any cause during the study period than were those who received the placebo.

And while the Finnish ATBC study failed to find a link between vitamin E and lung cancer, it did indicate that vitamin E may reduce the risk of prostate cancer by 34 percent.

Vitamin E and Cancer Treatment

Q: It looks like vitamin E hasn't been absolutely proven to reduce cancer risk. Does it have any promise as a cancer treatment?

A: Perhaps. Several studies indicate that vitamin E may help prevent the growth of tumors.

Q: In what way?

A: Test-tube studies have shown that vitamin E, working with prostaglandin E_2, may stop cancer cells from proliferating. Vitamin E has also been shown to reduce the growth of melanoma (a particularly deadly type of skin cancer) cells.

Q: Does it have any other effects?

A: In one test-tube study, vitamin E, along with vitamins C and A and beta carotene, increased the effectiveness of four drugs that inhibit cancer growth (*Nutrition and Cancer,* 1994). But evidence for vitamin E's cancer-treating ability remains inconclusive. In fact, there is some evidence that vitamin E may actually harm people with cancer.

Q: What evidence is that?

A: French researchers reported in 1995 that vitamin E may actually cause cancer to spread. The researchers studied 250 Italian women with breast cancer and found that those with larger, more aggressive or more invasive cancers had higher levels of vitamin E in their bodies. Similar results were reported in a small study of men and women with cancers at other sites (*Science News,* April 29, 1995).

Q: How could vitamin E encourage cancer growth?

A: Remember: Vitamin E can be either an antioxidant or a pro-oxidant, which in this case means that it might increase the oxidative damage associated with cancer. A review article published in the April 1996 *Journal of Nutrition* notes that this is particularly true when oxidative activity occurs in transformed cells, such as cancer cells.

Still, more studies indicate that vitamin E protects against cancer than indicate that it promotes cancer growth.

Q: That's good. But how exactly is vitamin E thought to protect against cancer?

A: There are several theories. As an antioxidant, vitamin E may protect our DNA—the genetic material that serves as a blueprint for normal cell division—from oxidative damage. When DNA is damaged, cells may divide in the uncontrolled way characteristic of cancer.

As a key player in the immune response, vitamin E may keep our immune system functioning well so that it can recognize and attack cancer cells.

Vitamin E may also prevent the formation of **nitrosamines**, substances formed in the digestive tract from the nitrates and nitrites we ingest. (Nitrates and nitrites, often used as food preservatives, are found in cured packaged meats such as bacon, cold cuts and hot dogs.) By blocking the formation of these substances, vitamin E may be able to block the formation of tumors that they could generate.

VITAMIN E AND THE NERVOUS SYSTEM

Q: You said that the evidence for vitamin E's ability to protect against cancer is not as great as for its heart-protective effects, and I see what you mean. What about its ability to protect the brain?

A: As we said in chapter 1, vitamin E appears to be crucial for the functioning of the nervous system, which, of course, includes the brain. While its exact role in the nervous system is unknown, deficiencies produce a number of neurological symptoms—symptoms that vitamin E has been shown to decrease. In addition, there is some evidence that vitamin E may help alleviate symptoms or slow the progression of several neurological disorders not linked to deficiencies, including Alzheimer's disease.

Q: What type of neurological symptoms is vitamin E deficiency thought to produce?

A: Vitamin E deficiency has been linked to unsteady gait, muscle weakness, abnormal eye movements, loss of reflexes and restricted field of vision.

Q: Those don't sound like neurological symptoms. What's their connection to the nervous system?

A: As you probably know, the brain is the nerve center of the entire body: It controls all bodily functions, including motor functions, balance, sensation, muscle strength, muscle control and coordination, as well as visual perception.

Q: I hadn't thought of that. Can vitamin E help alleviate neurological symptoms?

A: Several studies have found that vitamin E supplements or injections can alleviate neurological symptoms caused by vitamin E deficiency. Vitamin E supplements have also been used to prevent such symptoms in people with conditions that could make them susceptible to vitamin E deficiency.

Q: I know we discussed this before, but what conditions could lead to vitamin E deficiency?

A: Primarily conditions that affect the body's ability to absorb fats or vitamin E. These include cystic fibrosis, liver disorders, **pancreatitis** and **sprue**.

Q: What other neurological disorders is vitamin E thought to benefit?

A: Researchers have investigated vitamin E's effects on **Parkinson's disease**, **Huntington's disease**, **epilepsy** and **tardive dyskinesia**, as well as Alzheimer's disease.

Q: What have they found?

A: Several studies on Parkinson's disease, including a long-term study that tested the vitamin's effects against those of a placebo, have failed to find a benefit from vitamin E, but there is evidence that vitamin E may be of some benefit to people with the other conditions.

Q: OK. What effect does vitamin E have on Huntington's disease?

A: Vitamin E may slow the rate at which motor skills decline in Huntington's disease, a rare, inherited disease characterized by irregular, involuntary movements of the limbs and facial muscles and progressive dementia.

Q: What is that evidence?

A: In a study reported in the December 1995 *American Journal of Psychiatry,* researchers gave 73 people with Huntington's disease either vitamin E or a placebo and monitored the progression of their illness. While the vitamin treatment had no effect on overall neurological symptoms, it did have a therapeutic effect on the neurological symptoms of people who were in the early stages of the disease.

Q: To what did the researchers attribute vitamin E's effect?

A: To vitamin E's antioxidant properties. Evidence suggests that the degenerative neurological damage in Huntington's disease is caused by oxidation that kills brain cells.

Q: What about epilepsy?

A: In a Canadian study, vitamin E helped reduce the number of epileptic seizures in children. Earlier studies had shown that children with epilepsy have low levels of vitamin E.

Q: What about that other disease you mentioned, tardive dyskinesia? What kind of effect does vitamin E have on it, and why?

A: Tardive dyskinesia, a condition characterized by involuntary movement of the facial muscles and tongue, is a side effect of long-term use of tranquilizers prescribed to curb psychotic behavior. Because these drugs increase the production of free radicals in many parts of the body, including the part of the brain that regulates body movement, researchers have been studying the effects of vitamin E. The results of these studies show a beneficial effect. In an early study, doses of vitamin E between 400 and 1,200 I.U. per day resulted in a 43 percent reduction in involuntary movements. In a more recent study, large doses of vitamin E resulted in a 36 percent improvement (*American Journal of Psychiatry*, June 1994).

Q: What about Alzheimer's disease? What's the story there?

A: Only one study has looked at vitamin E's effect on Alzheimer's disease, but the results of that study raised hopes worldwide. Researchers from Columbia University, the University of California at San Diego and several other research centers reported in the April 24, 1997, *New England Journal of Medicine* that vitamin E in doses of 2,000 I.U. per day slowed the progression of Alzheimer's disease, an incurable illness that affects an estimated 4 million Americans.

Q: I want to know more about the study, but before we go into the details, why did the researchers select vitamin E?

A: Primarily because of the vitamin's antioxidant function. Alzheimer's disease is characterized by the death of brain cells, and there is some evidence that oxidation may contribute to their death. In one test-tube study, vitamin E stopped lipid peroxidation in brain cells and reduced cell death associated with a protein that has been linked to Alzheimer's disease.

Q: OK. Now back to the study: What exactly did the researchers find?

A: The researchers gave 341 people with moderately severe Alzheimer's disease vitamin E, an antioxidant medication called selegiline (Deprenyl) or a placebo for two years and monitored the amount of time it took for them to die, be institutionalized, lose the ability to perform at least two of three basic activities of daily living or have a worsening of their dementia. They found that both vitamin E and selegiline extended the amount of time until the study participants reached one of those milestones.

Q: What kind of an extension are we talking about?

A: While the people given the placebo took an average of 440 days to reach one of the study's endpoints, those given vitamin E took 670 days, and those given selegiline took 655 days. Those given both vitamin E and selegiline took 585 days to reach one of the study's endpoints.

Q: That doesn't seem very impressive. The people who took vitamin E only gained 230 days. Why was everyone so excited?

A: The number of days may not seem large, but it was a 52 percent gain. And the study focused on people whose disease was already moderately severe. Still, some experts have noted that the results of the study should be viewed cautiously.

Q: Why is that?

A: For several reasons. For starters, while vitamin E increased the amount of time until people with Alzheimer's disease reached one of the study endpoints, apparently slowing the progression of the disease, it had no effect on the disease's cognitive, or intellectual, symptoms.

In an editorial that accompanied the publication of the study, David A. Drachman, M.D., of the University of Massachusetts Medical Center in Worcester, and Paul Leber, M.D., of the U.S. Food and Drug Administration, questioned whether the endpoints of the study were appropriate. Death, they wrote, is not necessarily a direct consequence of Alzheimer's disease and rarely occurs before the other endpoints are reached; institutionalization is often related more to behavior than to impaired intellectual abilities; and even at the beginning of the study, 20 percent of the participants already needed assistance with one activity of daily living. The doctors questioned the vitamin's failure to affect scores on intellectual tests as well as the absence of an additional benefit when both drugs were administered together.

Even the researchers who conducted the study expressed some concern about the fact that the treatments failed to affect cognitive, or intellectual, functions. "The outcome of improved function despite the absence of improved cognition raises the possibility that the effect we observed is a nonspecific health benefit to which our primary outcome was sensitive," they wrote. In other words, vitamin E and selegiline might have actually affected something other than Alzheimer's disease itself.

Q: So what's the bottom line? Is vitamin E beneficial for people with Alzheimer's disease or not?

A: The bottom line is that more research is needed to determine the answer to that question.

"Our understanding of Alzheimer's disease suggests that its cause is multifactorial, with a cascade of degenerative events that may have many modifiable steps," Drachman and Leber wrote. "Antioxidants may someday be used as a part of a combined strategy to slow the course or even arrest the progress of Alzheimer's disease." Additional studies are needed, they wrote. But, they noted, since vitamin E is available over the counter, many caregivers may wish to try it.

While the Alzheimer's Association has not yet given the thumbs-up to vitamin E as a treatment for Alzheimer's disease, the American Psychiatric Association has included the vitamin, in doses between 200 and 800 I.U. per day, in its latest treatment guidelines for Alzheimer's disease.

> *"Compelling evidence from numerous basic research and epidemiological studies supports the notion that intakes of vitamin E above the RDA may be beneficial to maintain optimum health. However, results from limited intervention studies do not conclusively support this view."*
> —Mohsen Meydani, Ph.D.
> *Lancet,* January 21, 1995

VITAMIN E AND THE RESPIRATORY SYSTEM

Q: What effect does vitamin E have on the respiratory system?

A: As an antioxidant and a player in the immune response, vitamin E may protect the lungs from oxidative damage, including that caused by smoking and other pollutants.

Q: Is there any evidence that it does this?

A: Yes. Studies have found a link between vitamin E and lipid peroxidation in the lungs, and vitamin E has been shown to benefit lung function in smokers and people with asthma, as well as people without lung disorders.

Q: I'd like to know more. What is the link between vitamin E and lipid peroxidation?

A: In an animal study, Bulgarian researchers found that vitamin E levels in the lungs decrease and lipid peroxidation increases during times of stress (*Lung*, 1995).

Q: What does that mean?

A: It means that stress increases the need for vitamin E in the lungs. Remember: Antioxidants such as vitamin E are depleted when they neutralize free radicals.

Q: Do tobacco smoke and other pollutants also generate free radicals?

A: They certainly do. And several studies indicate that blood levels of vitamin E are lower in smokers than in nonsmokers. This could mean that the vitamin is being depleted as it protects the lungs from oxidative damage.

Q: I can understand how vitamin E may protect the lungs from oxidative damage, but is there any evidence that it does so?

A: There appears to be.

- Researchers evaluated whether taking antioxidant supplements, including 800 I.U. of vitamin E, 1,000 milligrams of vitamin C and 24 milligrams of beta carotene per day, had an effect on the exhaled ethane output (a measure of lipid peroxidation) of 10 smokers and three nonsmokers. They found that the average output decreased by 29 percent in smokers who took the supplements. This decrease translated into an improvement in a test that measures lung function, leading the researchers to conclude that antioxidants may lessen smoking-related lung injuries (*Chest*, July 1996).

- Researchers used a drug to induce inflammatory injury in rats. Twenty-four hours after they administered the drug, the researchers found increased levels of lipid peroxidation by-products in the lungs, along with decreased blood and tissue levels of vitamin E and swelling in the alveoli (tiny air sacs located at the tips of the lungs). When they gave the rats vitamin E, their blood levels of vitamin E increased and the degree of lung injury and lipid peroxidation slowed. The researchers concluded that vitamin E, given at the onset of a progressive inflammatory injury, can protect the lungs from oxidative damage and minimize the degree of lung injury (*Surgery,* February 1995).

- Vitamin E was shown to benefit mice with hypersensitivity pneumonitis, a disease characterized by an ongoing immune response in the lungs that results in oxidative damage (*Inflammation,* April 1995).

Q: What is vitamin E's connection to asthma?

A: At least one study has found that a high vitamin E intake—notably from food—may reduce the incidence of adult-onset asthma. The vitamin may also help improve breathing in people with the disease.

Q: First things first. What kind of risk reduction are we talking about?

A: Researchers who evaluated the diets and incidence of adult-onset asthma in 77,866 women over the course of 10 years found that those with the highest dietary intake of vitamin E were 47 percent less likely to develop asthma than were those who took in the least amount. The benefit was found from foods, not supplements (*American Journal of Respiratory and Critical Care Medicine,* May 1995).

Q: That's promising. Now, what can vitamin E do for people who already have asthma?

A: In a study presented at a 1997 meeting of the American Lung Association/American Thoracic Society, researchers from the University of Washington School of Public Health and Community Medicine in Seattle reported that adults with asthma given 400 I.U. of vitamin E and 500 milligrams of vitamin C had better lung function after being exposed to ozone (a reactive form of oxygen that acts as an air pollutant) during an exercise test than similar adults who were given a placebo.

Q: Didn't you say that vitamin E may also improve lung function in people without respiratory problems?

A: Yes. Researchers who compared the lung function of 2,633 adults with their dietary intake of vitamins E and C found that those who took in the most vitamin E performed better on two separate tests of lung function than did those who took in the least (*American Journal of Respiratory and Critical Care Medicine*, May 1995).

VITAMIN E AND THE EYES

Q: Moving right along, how is vitamin E thought to protect against cataracts?

A: Cataracts, the clouding of the eye's transparent lens, are thought to occur when proteins in the eye become oxidized, often as a result of sun exposure. Vitamin E, which is present in the eye, is thought to help protect the eye against this oxidative damage.

Q: Is there any evidence that it does this?

A: Yes. Test-tube and animal studies support this hypothesis, and several epidemiological studies indicate that it may hold true in people as well. Several studies have shown that people with high blood levels of vitamin E have a reduced risk of cataracts. But the research is not conclusive: Several studies have failed to show a benefit from vitamin E intake.

Q: I'd like specifics. What do these studies show?

A: According to a review article published in the December 1995 supplement of the *American Journal of Clinical Nutrition,* in one study, researchers measured the blood levels of 47 people with advanced cataracts and those of similar individuals with healthy eyes and followed them for a period of time. They found that those with vitamin E concentrations above a certain level had about one-half the rate of subsequent cataract surgery as those with E concentrations below that level. In another study that looked at vitamin E concentrations above and below a certain level, people with concentrations above the level were 48 percent less likely to have cataracts than were people with concentrations below the level. On the other hand, in two studies that looked at the use of vitamin E supplements, researchers found no link between vitamin E and cataract incidence or cataract surgery.

Q: Have there been any studies since then?

A: Yes. Several recent studies have looked at the link between vitamin E and cataracts.

- A study published in the *International Journal of Vitamin and Nutrition Research,* 1996), found that the levels of vitamin E in the lenses of people with cataracts were much lower than the levels of vitamin E in those people's blood.

- In a study published in the September 1996 *American Journal of Epidemiology,* researchers investigated the relationship between blood levels of vitamin E and early signs of cataracts in 410 Finnish men. They found that men who had the lowest blood levels of vitamin E were 3.7 times more likely to develop early signs of cataracts during the three-year study period than were those with the highest blood levels.

Q: Are there any other possible links between vitamin E and the eye?

A: Yes. Vitamin E has been proposed and used as a treatment for **retinopathy of prematurity (ROP)**, a condition developed by some premature infants in which abnormal blood vessels and scar tissue grow over the retina, often impairing vision. Because these infants, immediately after birth, are often placed in high-oxygen environments, some researchers theorize that oxidation may be responsible for the damage. Vitamin E has been proposed as a treatment because of its antioxidant properties and because some infants, particularly premature ones, have deficiencies.

Q: Is vitamin E effective in this context?

A: Study results are mixed, but two recent studies indicate some promise. In one study, premature infants with low birth weights treated with both vitamin E and cryotherapy, a surgical procedure to repair tears in the retina, had better visual outcomes after four years than those who received either treatment alone (*Journal of Pediatrics,* October 1995).

In another study, researchers who theorized that the discrepancies of earlier study results may be due to difficulty with getting vitamin E into the immature retina tested a water-soluble form of the vitamin in rats and found that it was effective in healing the retinal blood vessels (*Free Radical Biology and Medicine,* June 1997).

VITAMIN E AND THE SKIN

Q: I've heard that vitamin E is supposed to be of real benefit to the skin. What's the story?

A: Although vitamin E is an ingredient in many skin care products, claims that the vitamin prevents wrinkles and other aging-related skin problems remain unproven. And while there is some evidence that the vitamin may protect against ultraviolet radiation (and, hence, the sun's damaging effects on skin) and help scars and wounds heal, the studies are inconclusive.

Q: Let's start with the sun's effect on skin. Isn't that linked to cancer?

A: Yes. Ultraviolet radiation is linked to both cancer and skin aging. Because researchers think this damage may be caused by free radicals, there has been interest in studying whether vitamin E can offer a protective effect.

Q: What have the studies shown?

A: In one recent study, researchers found that topical application of tocopheryl sorbate, a form of vitamin E, decreased radiation-induced free radicals in the skin of hairless mice (*Journal of Investigative Dermatology*, April 1995).

Q: That sounds pretty promising. Has anyone looked at whether vitamin E offers any protection to human skin?

A: Yes, but with mixed results. While a review article published in the February 1996 *Dermatologic Surgery* found that an antioxidant compound that includes vitamin E reduced oxidative damage to skin cells exposed to ultraviolet light and toxic chemicals in test tubes and provided protection to humans exposed to ultraviolet light, researchers at Tufts and Boston universities found that vitamin E supplements did not appear to protect against sunburn caused by ultraviolet light. They gave 12 healthy volunteers either 400 I.U. of vitamin E per day or a placebo, then exposed their skin to ultraviolet light. There was no difference in the amount of ultraviolet light needed to induce redness or in the number of sunburned cells between the two groups. The researchers did note, however, that the dose of vitamin E they used increased blood levels of vitamin E by only 65 percent and did not increase skin tissue levels of the vitamin (*Archives of Dermatology,* October 1994).

Q: But that study used supplemental vitamin E rather than a topical form. Does that necessarily disprove the first study?

A: No. Clearly more research is needed to determine whether vitamin E—in either oral or topical form—can protect the skin from ultraviolet radiation and the damaging effects of sun exposure.

Q: What about scar and wound healing? Is the research in those departments any more conclusive?

A: Here, too, the results are mixed, although there has been more research on the subject.

- Italian researchers used either a traditional silicon gel treatment or a combination of silicon gel and vitamin E to treat problematic scars on 80 people. After two months, 95 percent of the people whose scars were treated with the vitamin E combination saw at least a 50 percent improvement in the color, size and cosmetic appearance of their scars, compared with 75 percent of the people whose scars were treated with silicon gel alone (*International Journal of Dermatology,* July 1995).

- A study reported in the June 1997 issue of *Ostomy Wound Management* found that topical application of essential fatty acids, including vitamin E, improved the moisture content and elasticity of skin and helped prevent the development of pressure sores in people with vitamin and mineral deficiencies.

- A review article published in the February 1996 *Dermatologic Surgery* reported that a commercial antioxidant compound that contains vitamin E helped facilitate the healing of infected and noninfected wounds in guinea pigs and rats.

- Israeli researchers reported that both topical and injected vitamin E decreased the healing time for laser burns in pigs (*Journal of Pharmaceutical Sciences,* August 1994).

- Triad, a commercial wound dressing that includes vitamin E, restored wound healing in rats whose wound healing was impaired by the drug doxorubicin (Doxo) (*American Surgeon,* June 1994).

- Researchers from the University of Miami Sylvester Comprehensive Cancer Center reported at a 1996 meeting of the American Society for Dermatological Surgery that vitamin E ointment applied to a wound after skin surgery was no more effective than ointments made from petrolatum and mineral oil or mineral oil alone in treating wounds. And several study participants reported allergic skin reactions to the vitamin treatment.

Q: I guess vitamin E hasn't actually earned its reputation as a miracle treatment for the skin, has it?

A: Not yet. In this matter, as in other matters relating to vitamin E, more research is needed.

VITAMIN E AND DIABETES

Q: What kind of reputation does vitamin E have as a treatment for diabetes?

A: A small but growing one. Researchers have long noted an association between vitamin E and diabetes. More recently, they have discovered that the vitamin may hold promise as a treatment to prevent several of the complications associated with the disease, which results from the body's inability to produce or use **insulin**, a hormone that enables the body to use sugar for energy.

Q: What is the association between vitamin E and diabetes?

A: Vitamin E levels in the blood of people with diabetes are generally lower than levels found in people who don't have diabetes, which suggests that the disease either increases the demand for vitamin E or alters its use.

Q: Does this translate into an increased risk?

A: It appears so. In a recent study, researchers followed 944 Finnish men for four years. These men had relatively low blood levels of vitamin E, and 60 percent took in less than 10 milligrams of the vitamin a day. When the researchers looked at their poor nutritional status, along with other risk factors, they determined that low vitamin E levels raised the risk of developing diabetes nearly fourfold (*British Medical Journal,* October 28, 1995).

Q: Are there any other connections between vitamin E and diabetes?

A: Yes. Some studies indicate that low dietary intakes of vitamin E might alter blood sugar, or glucose, levels and that adequate intakes might help reduce blood sugar levels. Vitamin E may also reduce levels of insulin and triglycerides, fatty compounds in the blood that are present in high levels in many people with diabetes.

Q: Have there been any recent studies on these connections?

A: Yes.

- In a study of 30 elderly people with heart disease (a disease that often goes hand-in-hand with diabetes), supplementation with 900 I.U. of vitamin E per day for three months was shown to lower concentrations of insulin and triglycerides in the blood (*American Journal of Clinical Nutrition,* April 1995).

- Researchers who gave 35 people with type-1 diabetes (in which the body loses the capacity to produce insulin) either 100 I.U. of vitamin E per day or a placebo found that the vitamin decreased triglyceride and blood sugar levels (*Journal of the American College of Nutrition,* October 1995).

- Italian researchers reported in two separate studies published in the *American Journal of Clinical*

Nutrition (May 1993 and June 1994) that vitamin E supplements, in doses of 900 I.U. or more, improved the body's ability to use insulin to metabolize blood sugar.

Q: Are these the only mechanisms by which vitamin E may benefit people with diabetes?

A: No. Recent research has also focused on vitamin E's antioxidant capabilities and its ability to inhibit protein kinase C, the enzyme that encourages the proliferation of smooth muscle cells.

Q: What do those have to do with diabetes? I thought they were connected to atherosclerosis.

A: They are. People with diabetes are at increased risk of atherosclerosis and, consequently, heart disease and stroke. There is some evidence that LDL is more easily oxidized in people with diabetes. And protein kinase C, which is linked to atherosclerosis, is also linked to high blood sugar, which may play a role in oxidation.

Q: Is there any evidence that vitamin E can help counter these complications associated with diabetes?

A: Yes.

- Researchers from the University of Texas Southwestern Medical Center in Dallas gave 28 people with diabetes either 1,200 I.U. of vitamin E or a placebo daily for eight weeks. Those who received the supplements had higher levels of vitamin E in their blood and in their LDL; their LDL also showed a reduction in its susceptibility to oxidation (*American Journal of Clinical Nutrition,* May 1996).

- A study reported in *Diabetes Care* (June 1995) found that men with type-2 diabetes (in which the body produces insulin, but that insulin is ineffective) who took 1,600 I.U. of vitamin E per day for 10 weeks increased their blood and LDL levels of vitamin E approximately fourfold and saw a decreased susceptibility of their LDL to oxidation.
- Researchers found that vitamin E decreased elevated protein kinase C activity in the cells of blood vessels in people with diabetes (*Diabetes*, July 1996).

OTHER VITAMIN E USES

Q: It sounds like vitamin E may be of real benefit to people with diabetes. Are there any other conditions that it might benefit?

A: In recent years, researchers have found connections between vitamin E and muscle function and between vitamin E and several health problems unique to women. Several studies have also linked the vitamin to **rheumatoid arthritis**, liver function and fertility. Vitamin E supplements are also used to treat diseases that are caused by vitamin E deficiencies, such as hemolytic anemia, and diseases that often result in vitamin E deficiencies such as cystic fibrosis, liver cirrhosis, pancreatic insufficiency and sprue.

Vitamin E and Muscle Function

Q: Let's start with the muscles. What links have been found between vitamin E and muscle function?

A: Researchers at Pennsylvania State University and Tufts University have found that vitamin E may help reduce postexercise muscle damage—particularly in sedentary individuals or people who do not exercise often.

Q: Wait a minute. I thought exercise was good for muscles. How can it damage them, and what can vitamin E do to help?

A: Vigorous exercise increases the need for and use of oxygen, which, as you know, is often responsible for oxidative reactions. The increased oxygen consumption during exercise generates free radicals that can damage fats, which are present in both the blood and cell membranes. Vitamin E is thought to protect the fats in blood and cell membranes from that oxidative damage.

Q: I see. Now, let's get back to the research. What exactly did the researchers find?

A: In a 1995 study, they gave sedentary men either 800 I.U. of vitamin E or a placebo for 48 days and found that those given vitamin produced fewer by-products of lipid peroxidation when they exercised than did those given the placebo.

Q: Have any other studies found that vitamin E has a protective effect on muscles?

A: Yes. William J. Evans, Ph.D., a Pennsylvania State University professor who serves on the U.S. Olympic Committee that reviews dietary supplements for athletes, reported that vitamin E may help repair microscopic tears in muscles that cause muscle soreness in people unaccustomed to exercise. Evans theorized that in addition to decreasing the production of damaging free radicals, vitamin E may help mobilize immune system cells to invade the damaged muscle and initiate repair (*Internal Medicine News,* July 15, 1996).

Vitamin E and Women's Health

Q: What conditions unique to women is vitamin E thought to benefit?

A: There is some evidence—although inconclusive—that vitamin E can benefit women with **fibrocystic breast disease** and ease premenstrual symptoms.

Q: What is fibrocystic breast disease, and what is its connection to vitamin E?

A: Fibrocystic breast disease is a common condition characterized by lumps in the breast. Although these lumps are generally harmless, women with fibrocystic breast disease may be at greater risk of breast cancer. In several studies, vitamin E provided some relief from fibrocystic breast disease. In the most widely cited study, 22 of 26 women improved after they took 600 I.U. of vitamin E daily for eight weeks. But in another study, women who took vitamin E had no more relief than women who took a placebo.

More recently, Indian researchers reported that vitamin E treatment provided relief to 41 percent of women with benign breast disease who received the treatment. While this rate was lower than the rate of women who found relief from the drug danazol (Danocrine), few of the women treated with vitamin E reported side effects, while one-third of the women treated with danazol did (*Journal of the Indian Medical Association*, January 1997).

Q: What about premenstrual symptoms?

A: In two older, small studies, vitamin E in doses between 300 and 600 I.U. provided some relief from certain premenstrual symptoms.

Vitamin E and Rheumatoid Arthritis

Q: You said that vitamin E has been linked to rheumatoid arthritis. In what way?

A: Several studies have linked low blood levels of vitamin E with an increased risk of rheumatoid arthritis, an inflammatory disease of the joints that is thought to result when the immune system attacks the body's own tissues.

Q: What exactly did those studies find?

A: In one study, reported in the June 1994 *Veris,* Finnish researchers measured the blood levels of vitamin E and other antioxidants in more than 1,400 adults and followed them for 20 years. They found that those with the lowest concentrations of antioxidants in their blood were 8.3 percent more likely to develop rheumatoid arthritis during the study period than were those with the highest concentrations.

In another study, researchers compared the blood levels of vitamin E and other antioxidants in 21 people with rheumatoid arthritis, six people with lupus (an autoimmune disease) and 108 healthy people. They found that those with rheumatoid arthritis and lupus had lower blood levels of vitamin E, vitamin A and beta carotene than those without the diseases (*Annals of Rheumatic Diseases,* May 1997).

Vitamin E and Liver Function

Q: What is vitamin E's link to liver function?

A: Studies have shown that blood levels of vitamin E are low in people with three diseases that affect the liver—**hemochromatosis**, alcoholic liver disease and **Wilson's disease**. And German researchers reported in 1996 that blood levels of vitamin E may also be low in people with viral **hepatitis**.

Q: Do the experts have any idea why the levels are low?

A: The German researchers who found low blood levels of vitamin E in people with viral hepatitis suggest that free radical damage may play a role in the disease and suggested that vitamin E might help treat it (*Free Radical Research,* December 1996).

Similarly, free radical theory has been used to explain the low levels of vitamin E in people with alcoholic liver disease, but a recent study indicates that the vitamin may not be an effective treatment for the disease. When Chilean researchers gave 67 people with cirrhosis either 500 milligrams of vitamin E or a placebo each day for a year, they found that the vitamin had no significant effect on liver function, hospitalization rates or mortality (*Journal of the American College of Nutrition,* April 1995).

Vitamin E and Fertility

Q: I've heard that vitamin E helps boost the sex drive. Is it true?

A: Vitamin E's alleged ability to boost the sex drive appears to be a myth—spurred, perhaps, by early research that found that the vitamin played a crucial role in animal reproductive systems. It does not appear to play the same role in the human reproductive system, but there is some evidence that vitamin E may play a role in fertility.

Q: How is vitamin E linked to fertility?

A: Vitamin E may help protect the integrity of sperm and improve their mobility, which could improve fertility.

- In one study, researchers gave vitamin E and selenium supplements to nine men with fertility problems related to their sperm. They found that the vitamins improved sperm motility, the percentage of living sperm and the percentage of normal sperm in the men, although none of their partners reported a pregnancy during the study (*Biological Trace Elements Research,* Summer 1996).

- Another study examined the effect of vitamin E supplements on 15 men with normal, functioning sperm who had low fertilization rates. After receiving 200 milligrams of vitamin E daily for three months, the men saw an increase in their fertilization rate (*Fertility and Sterility,* September 1996).

PUTTING IT ALL TOGETHER

Q: Now that we've gone through all the research, I'm still confused. While some of the research indicates that vitamin E has some real health benefits, some of it doesn't. Why the discrepancy?

A: There are a number of possible reasons. One of the primary reasons involves the research itself. Investigators use a variety of techniques, and these various techniques often result in conflicting results. This is perfectly normal—in fact, these differing findings are necessary to test theories and build consensus among research findings.

Q: In what way?

A: Research that shows a link between something may be intriguing and may hint at a cause and effect, but by no means does it prove the link. While people with diabetes, cancer or several other diseases often have lower blood levels of vitamin E than healthy individuals, it does not necessarily mean that these diseases are caused by a lack of vitamin E or that increasing vitamin E intake will provide a benefit. Studies may link high vitamin E intake to lower risk of heart disease, but they do not prove that vitamin E actually prevents heart disease. To prove cause and effect, more research is needed.

Q: What kind of research?

A: The kind that isolates the effects of vitamin E from the effects of other substances and compares those effects with the effects of a placebo. Without this type of research, theories remain theories. They may accumulate more supporting evidence, but they remain unproven. This is why public health officials have not yet advised people to take vitamin E supplements to prevent heart disease, although many take them themselves.

Q: I guess I can understand that caution to some extent—especially for conditions for which the research is conflicting. But there seems to be a lot of that conflicting research. How should I interpret it?

A: Be aware of the research findings to date and keep track of new findings as they emerge. You may have already drawn some conclusions about vitamin E's various health benefits, or you may need more information before you can do so. And your conclusion, like the research findings themselves, may change in the future.

3 WHAT ELSE DO I NEED TO KNOW?

Q: Even if only a few of the claims made for vitamin E are ultimately substantiated, am I right in assuming that the vitamin is pretty important to our health and well-being?

A: Yes. In fact, it's already been proven that vitamin E is necessary for the body to function normally—that's why it's been labeled a vitamin.

DOSAGE

Q: How much vitamin E do we need to stay healthy and prevent disease?

A: You're asking two different questions. As you may recall from the preceding chapters, the amounts recommended to stay healthy—in other words, to prevent deficiency-related symptoms—are much lower than the amounts that have been linked to disease prevention.

Q: OK. I'll break up my question. How much vitamin E do we need to stay healthy?

A: As we said in chapter 1, the Recommended Dietary Allowance (RDA) for vitamin E is 15 international units (I.U.), or 10 milligrams tocopherol equivalents (TE), for adult men and 12 I.U., or 8 milligrams TE, for women. RDAs for other groups range from 3 milligrams TE for infants to 12 milligrams TE for breast-feeding women in their first six months of lactation. The chart that follows gives the daily RDAs for all gender and age-groups.

Recommended Dietary Allowances for Vitamin E

Category	Age	Amount in milligrams TE
Infants	0-5 months	3
	5 months-1 year	4
Children	1-3 years	6
	4-10 years	7
Men	11+ years	10
Women	11+ years	8
	Pregnant	10
	Lactating (1st 6 months)	12
	Lactating (2nd 6 months)	11

Q: Refresh my memory. What exactly do these recommendations mean, and what is a tocopherol equivalent? Is it different than an international unit?

A: Tocopherol equivalents and international units are arbitrary measurements that enable us to compare and measure different forms of vitamin E. (As you may recall, the different forms of vitamin E have varying levels of biological activity in the body.) The international unit, which is used as a measure for both vitamin E and vitamin A, is a unit of measure unto itself. The tocopherol equivalent, which is used solely to measure vitamin E, is often measured in milligrams. Although both measurement units are designed to enable different forms of the vitamin to be compared, the measurement units cannot be compared with one another. One I.U. of vitamin E is equal to 1 milligram of synthetic alpha-tocopherol. One milligram TE is equal to 1.49 I.U. of natural alpha-tocopherol.

> *One tablespoon of wheat germ oil provides 28.3 I.U. of vitamin E; walnut oil, 13.1 I.U.; sunflower oil, 10.3 I.U.; cottonseed oil, 8.9 I.U.; safflower oil, 8.5 I.U.; and corn oil, 3.6 I.U.*

Q: That answers one part of my question. Now, to the other part: What exactly do those RDA recommendations mean?

A: The RDAs are levels of nutrient intake—from either foods or supplements—that the National Academy of Sciences' Food and Nutrition Board believes to be adequate to meet the known nutrient needs of practically all healthy people.

RDAs go somewhat beyond what is needed to prevent deficiency-related diseases—in fact, it's possible to consistently take in less than the RDA for a particular nutrient and not suffer adverse health problems as a result. On the other hand, amounts higher than the RDA may be necessary for optimal health.

Q: Before we go any further, could you list the deficiency symptoms of vitamin E once again?

A: Certainly. In infants, the symptoms include irritability, fluid retention and anemia. In adults, lethargy, apathy, inability to concentrate, loss of balance, staggering gait and anemia are deficiency-related symptoms. Hemorrhage is also possible because vitamin E is important in maintaining red blood cells.

Q: And the RDAs are designed to prevent these symptoms. But didn't you say in chapter 1 that the RDAs are undergoing review?

A: Yes. The Food and Nutrition Board is in the process of revising the RDAs so that they will take into consideration not only the amount of each nutrient that is needed to prevent deficiency diseases but also the amount needed to decrease the risk of chronic diseases such as heart disease and cancer. These revised RDAs will become part of a new set of recommendations known as Dietary Reference Intakes (DRIs).

Q: When will the DRIs for vitamin E be available?

A: The Food and Nutrition Board hopes to establish DRIs for all essential nutrients by the year 2000, but it has not yet established a precise time frame for the release of the new recommendations.

Q: In the meantime, how do we know how much vitamin E we need to reduce our risk of chronic disease and reap the vitamin's full benefits?

A: The answer depends on whom you ask.
Vitamin E proponents have recommended dosages ranging anywhere from 100 to 1,200 I.U. per day to help maintain health and combat chronic illnesses. Those who are more skeptical of vitamin E's abilities, those who are fearful of its pro-oxidant tendencies and those who fear potential side effects from large doses generally recommend doses closer to the RDA. Others recommend levels somewhere in between.

Q: Why such a discrepancy?

A: For two primary reasons: The one universal recommendation we have—the RDA—does not address this optimal amount; and, as you saw in chapter 2, studies on vitamin E's protective effects cover a wide range of dosages. Some studies indicate that vitamin E confers health benefits at levels near the RDA; others have found benefits only at much higher levels.

Q: Does the level at which health benefits are found differ according to the specific condition or according to the way the study is conducted?

A: Both. Some studies that have examined vitamin E's health benefits have simply compared the vitamin E intake of study participants; much of this research has found that those who take in the most vitamin E appear to benefit more than those who take in the least. Some studies have focused on the amount of vitamin E people take in through food, while others have examined the effects of supplements in a variety of specified doses. These differing study protocols do translate into differing findings.

But the condition, too, seems to play a role. While small doses of vitamin E—doses near the RDA—have been found in some studies to confer protection against cancer or to boost immune function, larger doses appear to be needed to confer protection against heart disease. Most of the studies that have indicated that vitamin E protects the heart have found such a benefit only in doses of 100 I.U. of more.

Q: No wonder it's difficult to determine an optimal amount! Do any other factors figure in here?

A: Yes. Studies show that a person's vitamin E needs also depend on his ability to absorb fat, his diet and his lifestyle.

Q: I know we discussed a person's ability to absorb fat earlier, but I need a memory refresher. What exactly does that have to do with vitamin E?

A: People who have difficulty absorbing fat also have difficulty absorbing vitamin E, which is fat soluble. These people, including premature, low birth weight infants, people with chronic liver disease or disorders of the pancreas and people with cystic fibrosis, are at higher risk of developing a vitamin E deficiency. People who eat very low-fat diets, too, may be at risk.

Q: Why is that?

A: Because the body needs some fat in the diet to absorb vitamin E.

One-half cup of shelled sunflower seeds contains nearly 40 I.U. of vitamin E, along with 35 grams of fat.

Q: Do any other dietary habits affect vitamin E needs?

A: Yes. People who take in large amounts of polyunsaturated fat—the type of fat found in vegetable oils and margarines—may require more vitamin E in their diets.

Q: Why?

A: Because a large intake of polyunsaturated fat increases the amount of polyunsaturated fat in body tissues and, consequently, the amount of vitamin E needed to protect those tissue fats from oxidation.

Q: Wait a minute. Aren't foods that are high in polyunsaturated fats also high in vitamin E?

A: Although some of the foods that are high in polyunsaturated fat are relatively high in vitamin E, not all are. And some of the foods that do contain vitamin E contain one of the less potent forms of the vitamin. Corn and soybean oils, for example, are rich in **gamma-tocopherol**, which has one-tenth the biological activity of alpha-tocopherol. (New research does indicate, however, that gamma-tocopherol may be effective in preventing degenerative diseases.) Thus, the source of the food, as well as its polyunsaturated fat content, comes into play in determining vitamin E needs.

Q: Do any other dietary factors figure into that equation?

A: Yes. Intake of other antioxidants may also play a role in vitamin E requirements because antioxidants interact with one another. Vitamin C, for example, is thought to restore vitamin E to its active antioxidant form after vitamin E has been rendered inactive in an oxidative reaction. Thus, a high intake of vitamin C could, theoretically, reduce the need for vitamin E. But because this interaction has not yet been fully confirmed and because vitamin E's relation to other antioxidants also remains unclear, the exact role other antioxidants play in determining individual vitamin E needs remains unknown.

Q: Didn't you say that lifestyle factors also have an effect on an individual's vitamin E needs?

A: Yes. Exercise, smoking, alcohol use and exposure to air pollution all may increase oxidative stress, thus increasing the body's need for vitamin E and other antioxidants. As we noted in chapter 2, smokers often have lower blood levels of vitamin E than nonsmokers. And vitamin E supplements appear to reduce oxidative damage in people who exercise.

Pregnancy also increases vitamin E requirements—in large part because the nutrient status of mothers affects the nutrient status of newborns. Studies show that blood levels of vitamin E in fetuses parallel those of their mothers, but at lower concentrations. As a result, many researchers speculate that increasing vitamin E intake during pregnancy may increase vitamin E levels in newborns, thus preventing anemia and other deficiency-related symptoms.

TOXICITY

Q: I never thought so many factors went into determining how much of a nutrient we need for adequate health. No wonder it's difficult to determine how much we need. But does anyone need **megadoses** of vitamin E?

A: That depends on what you mean by the word megadose. Some people use the word to define large doses or doses that exceed recommendations. In scientific terms, however, it has been defined as a dose that is 10 times the RDA or more. In the case of vitamin E, this would be a dose that is 120 I.U., or 80 milligrams TE, or more for women or 150 I.U., or 100 milligrams TE, or more for men—rather small in comparison with the high doses advocated by some people and the amounts used in many vitamin E studies. For example, many of the studies on vitamin E's heart-protective properties have found benefits from doses of 400 I.U. or more. Clearly, in those instances, megadoses proved beneficial. But as to whether or not anyone actually needs megadoses, as defined scientifically, that remains to be seen.

Q: Are megadoses harmful?

A: Vitamin E is considered relatively safe, even in large doses. That said, however, experts caution about megadoses, which have been linked in some people to an increased tendency to bleed and, according to informal reports, to an increased risk of blood clots. Other signs of toxicity include fatigue, nausea, muscle weakness, stomach upset and skin disorders. Anyone who experiences these symptoms while taking large doses of vitamin E should discontinue use. Anyone experiencing bleeding disorders while taking high doses of vitamin E should consult her doctor.

DRUG INTERACTIONS

Q: Speaking of bleeding, didn't you say in chapter 2 that people taking certain drugs shouldn't take vitamin E?

A: Yes. Because of vitamin E's anticoagulant properties, people who are taking anticoagulant drugs such as warfarin (Coumadin) or people who have a known vitamin K deficiency should take vitamin E supplements only under a doctor's supervision.

Q: Does vitamin E interact with any other drugs?

A: Yes. While the interaction between vitamin E and anticoagulant drugs is the most well known, several other drugs may decrease blood levels of vitamin E or increase vitamin E requirements. According to Joe and Teresa Graedon, authors of *The People's Guide to Deadly Drug Interactions,* these drugs include oral contraceptives and hormone replacement therapy, which may lower blood levels of vitamin E, and mineral oil laxatives and cholesterol medications such as colestid and questran, which can interfere with the absorption of fats and fat-soluble vitamins.

NUTRIENT INTERACTIONS

Q: What about other nutrients? Does vitamin E interact with them in any way?

A: Yes. And we must stress that these interactions are, in some instances, positive. For example, as we've said, vitamin C may donate electrons to vitamin E after vitamin E has donated its own electrons to free radicals in an attempt to neutralize an oxidative reaction. This restores vitamin E's antioxidant power, enabling it to continue its efforts to neutralize free radicals. Because vitamin C may regenerate vitamin E, it may, theoretically, reduce the need for vitamin E.

> *Vitamin E acts as an antioxidant in foods, particularly vegetable oils. It keeps the oils from oxidizing and turning rancid.*

Q: Didn't you say that the need for vitamin E may also relate to intake of other antioxidants?

A: Yes. Several studies indicate that beta carotene, in doses between 15 and 60 milligrams per day, lowers blood levels of vitamin E, but other, more recent studies have failed to find a link between beta carotene intake and blood levels of vitamin E. And one recent study indicates that increasing dietary intake of vitamin E, vitamin C or carotenoids (including beta carotene) may boost blood levels of one or both of the other antioxidants, a finding that suggests that the antioxidants work together to protect the body from oxidation.

The latter study, reported in the December 1995 *American Journal of Clinical Nutrition,* found that in people over age 60, those whose diets contained at least 220 milligrams of vitamin C had 18 percent more vitamin E in their blood than did those who ate less than 120 milligrams of vitamin C—even after the researchers corrected for vitamin E intake. Vitamin E intake above 30 milligrams per day also increased blood levels of vitamin C, and increased intake of carotenoids appeared to raise blood levels of vitamin E—a finding that contradicts the earlier studies on vitamin E and beta carotene. Clearly, more research is needed to determine whether vitamin E should be taken in conjunction with beta carotene.

SUPPLEMENTS

Q: I'm considering boosting my intake of vitamin E with supplements. What's out there?

A: Quite a bit. Individual vitamin E supplements are available in a number of forms, brands and doses. Vitamin E is also available in combination with other nutrients—as part of a multivitamin and mineral supplement or an antioxidant supplement, for example.

Q: I'm not very familiar with multivitamin and mineral supplements. What type of vitamins and minerals do they contain and in what amounts?

A: Multivitamin and mineral supplements contain any number of vitamins and minerals in varying doses. Most contain some, but not all, of the nutrients for which RDAs have been established, in varying amounts. They may also contain varying amounts of nutrients for which no RDA has been established.

Q: What type of multivitamin and mineral supplement do the experts recommend?

A: While not all nutrition experts advocate nutritional supplements, many do believe that a multivitamin and mineral supplement can serve as "insurance" that you are getting enough of the essential vitamins and minerals. These experts generally suggest that you buy a supplement that provides 100 percent of the RDA of the nutrients that have an RDA.

Q: Do any multivitamin and mineral supplements contain more than the RDA of certain nutrients?

A: Yes. Some do offer high amounts of antioxidants such as vitamins E and C and beta carotene. But it is easy enough, and sometimes cheaper, to simply purchase individual supplements of these vitamins.

Q: I'd like to know more about individual vitamin E supplements. In what forms are they available?

A: Vitamin E comes in a variety of forms. As we've said, eight different substances have vitamin E activity, including alpha-, beta-, delta- and gamma-tocopherol. Alpha-tocopherol is the most active and appears most often in supplements. But the other forms may also appear in supplements—often together, if the supplement is marketed as having mixed tocopherols.

Q: But since alpha-tocopherol is the most active form, isn't it best to look for it?

A: Not necessarily. Because all of the naturally occurring forms of vitamin are present in foods, some experts recommend that people using supplements choose those with mixed tocopherols, which may more accurately reflect the manner in which the body would obtain vitamin E from foods. And new research shows that gamma-tocopherol may be as effective as alpha-tocopherol in preventing degenerative diseases (*Science News,* April 5, 1997).

Q: Is there any difference between natural and synthetic vitamin E?

A: Yes. Natural vitamin E is derived from natural sources, often soybean oil, while synthetic vitamin E, like other synthetic vitamins, is constructed from organic molecules found in a wide array of substances. The natural form has slightly more biological activity in the body than the synthetic form.

Q: Does that mean the natural form is better?

A: Because natural vitamin E is more potent than the synthetic version, many people swear by it. Indeed, sales of natural vitamin E have been skyrocketing in recent years, topping 25 percent of all vitamin E consumption in

1995 alone (*Chemical Marketing Reporter,* August 7, 1995). But this does not necessarily mean that synthetic vitamin E is inferior to the natural form. Manufacturers of synthetic vitamin E supplements compensate for their products' lower potency by increasing the amount of vitamin E they put into their supplements until they equal the potency of natural supplements. Thus, a synthetic vitamin E supplement that contains 400 I.U. of vitamin E should have the same potency as a natural vitamin E supplement that contains 400 I.U. of vitamin E.

That said, however, some experts still prefer vitamin E in its natural form.

Q: Why is that?

A: For several reasons: The amount of vitamin E added to synthetic supplements is standardized based on information gleaned from animal studies, rather than studies of humans. At least one human study suggests that the currently accepted ratio of **bioavailability** between natural and synthetic vitamin E is greater than originally thought. In other words, it may take more of the synthetic form than originally thought to equal the potency of the natural form. In addition, both animal and human studies suggest that the natural form of vitamin E remains in body tissues longer than the synthetic form.

Q: So, what's the bottom line? Should I opt for the natural form or the synthetic form?

A: That's a matter of personal preference. The natural form may be slightly more potent than the synthetic form, but most of the studies that suggest vitamin E may help protect the heart have used the cheaper, synthetic form.

Q: How can I tell if the supplement I'm buying is natural or synthetic?

A: Read the label. Vitamin E supplements invariably bear the hyphenated name of the form of the vitamin on the label. When the vitamin name begins with d- or RRR-, the supplement contains a natural form of vitamin E; when the name begins with dl- or all-rac-, it contains a synthetic form.

Q: That sounds easy enough. But now I'm curious. What are the other parts of the hyphenated name, and what do they mean?

A: The second part of the hyphenated name tells you what form of vitamin E you are getting—alpha, beta, delta or gamma—while the third part indicates whether the alpha compound has been chemically isolated from the other three tocopherols by a special chemical procedure. If the alpha compound has been isolated, the final part of the hyphenated name will end in -yl, if it has not been isolated, the name end in -ol. Thus, you end up with names such as d-alpha-tocopherol or dl-alpha-tocopheryl.

Some forms of vitamin E also contain a fourth name, which indicates that the vitamin has been combined with another compound to improve its stability. In liquids, this compound is generally acetate; in tablets and dry capsules, the compound is generally succinate.

Q: So what are some of the forms of vitamin E that are widely available?

A: The most common include d-alpha-tocopherol, d-alpha-tocopheryl acetate, d-alpha-tocopheryl succinate, dl-alpha-tocopherol, dl-alpha-tocopheryl acetate and dl-alpha-tocopheryl succinate. And as we said, there are also supplements that contain mixed tocopherols. These include all four tocopherols—alpha, beta, delta and gamma.

Q: We've talked about the form of vitamin E included in supplements, but what about the forms of the supplements themselves? Do they come in pill form?

A: Yes. Vitamin E supplements are available in pills, capsules, tablets and oral solutions in a variety of doses.

Q: Which is best?

A: That's primarily a matter of personal preference. Size, taste and ability to swallow may make one form preferable over the others.

Q: What about the manufacturer? Should I go for the name brand, or is the store brand OK?

A: Many store brands are similar in formulation to expensive brand-name vitamins, but they cost much less. Check labels to see what you are getting for your money and compare. If a manufacturer claims its product is more readily absorbed or better balanced, you may want to contact the company and ask for research that backs up such marketing claims.

Q: Speaking about absorption, is there any way I can tell if the supplements I'm buying will dissolve properly and be absorbed?

A: Look for the letters "U.S.P." on the label. This means that the supplement meets manufacturing standards set by the U.S. Pharmacopoeia, an independent, nonprofit organization that sets standards for strength, quality, purity, packaging and labeling for medical products used in the United States.

You can also help your body absorb the nutrients in a supplement by taking it at the end of a meal. The digestive juices stimulated by food help the supplement break down and be absorbed. And when taking a fat-soluble vitamin such as vitamin E, remember to include a little fat in your meal.

Q: Is there any way I can make sure that the supplement I'm buying is fresh and at full potency?

A: There's no way to be absolutely certain. Some supplement labels contain expiration dates beyond which you should not buy the product. Look for these dates. If no dates appear, look instead for a product that has good outer and inner seals.

Q: How should I store my supplements?

A: Keep your supplements in an opaque container rather than a clear one, and store the container in a dry, dark place away from sunlight and heat, making sure the lid is tightly sealed. Air, sunlight and dampness can affect the potency of vitamin supplements.

DIETARY SOURCES

Q: What about the vitamin E found in foods? Is it any better than the vitamin E found in supplements?

A: As we mentioned, natural vitamin E is more potent than synthetic vitamin E, but it is very difficult to obtain large amounts of vitamin E from food alone, especially if you follow the healthy eating guidelines established by the government and other health advisory groups.

Q: Refresh my memory. In which foods is vitamin E found?

A: The richest dietary sources include wheat germ; soybean, cotton seed, peanut, corn, hazelnut, sunflower and almond oils; whole grain cereals; eggs; mayonnaise; and whole, raw seeds and nuts, as well as fortified cereals.

> *Brown rice is the only form of rice that contains vitamin E.*

Q: Which of these do we get most of our vitamin E from?

A: Vegetable oils are the major dietary source of vitamin E in the developed world; grain products, including fortified cereals, and fruits and vegetables also provide significant amounts of vitamin E.

Q: Which form of vitamin E is most common in foods?

A: All forms of vitamin E are contained in foods, which is one reason some experts recommend mixed tocopherol supplements. That said, however, alpha-tocopherol is the most widely available form found in food, primarily because it has the most biological activity. It is the dominant tocopherol in olive, canola, safflower and sunflower oils, while gamma-tocopherol is the dominant form in corn and soybean oils.

Q: Do most people get enough vitamin E?

A: It depends on what you mean by enough. According to a U.S. Department of Agriculture survey, the average vitamin E intake for women 19 to 50 years old was less than 90 percent of the RDA, although men of the same age averaged intakes close to 100 percent of the RDA, so by that standard, at least half the population is getting enough vitamin E. But most people are only taking in about half of the 30 I.U. recommended by the government on food labels.

Q: Is it possible to get 30 I.U. from food alone without sacrificing a low-fat diet?

A: Yes. Particularly if you add fortified cereals to your diet. Most of these cereals contain at least 40 percent of the Reference Daily Intake, or Daily Value, the amount shown on food labels.

Q: Is there any way to maximize the amount of vitamin E we get from foods?

A: Yes. Because vitamin E can be lost from foods during cooking, processing or storage, use unprocessed products such as unmilled grains and cold-pressed or unrefined vegetable oils whenever possible, store vitamin E-rich foods in airtight containers and avoid exposing them to light.

Q: Is there anything else I need to know about vitamin E?

A: We've covered the basics. But as you know, new information on health and nutrition becomes available every day. Be alert to new findings on the role vitamin E plays in the body, the vitamin's potential health benefits and new dosage recommendations to keep yourself up-to-date on this popular and beneficial nutrient.

> *The following foods provide 20 percent or more of the RDA of vitamin E in a 3½ ounce serving: almonds, asparagus, duck, goose, kale, spinach, prunes, sunflower seeds.*

GLOSSARY

Alpha-tocopherol: The most biologically active form of vitamin E.

Alpha-tocopheroxyl radical: An unstable, oxidized form of vitamin E thought to have pro-oxidant properties.

Alzheimer's disease: A progressive, degenerative brain disease that impairs memory, thinking and behavior.

Anemia: A decrease in red blood cells that reduces the blood's ability to carry oxygen; symptoms include fatigue, dizziness, headache, insomnia and pale skin.

Angina: Severe chest pain caused by an insufficient amount of oxygen-rich blood being supplied to the heart muscle.

Antibodies: Substances made by the immune system to neutralize antigens.

Anticoagulant: A substance that suppresses, delays or prevents the coagulation of blood.

Antigens: Substances foreign to the body that cause the immune system to form antibodies to neutralize them.

Antioxidant: A substance with the ability to interfere with oxygen-generated, or oxidative, reactions. Antioxidants neutralize free radicals, unstable atomic or molecular fragments that can damage cells. Nutrients that act as antioxidants include vitamins C and E, beta carotene and selenium.

Atherosclerosis: A condition in which the inner layers of the artery walls become thick and irregular due to deposits of fat, cholesterol and other substances.

Autoimmune diseases: Diseases caused by the action of the immune system against the body; they occur because the immune cells can't differentiate between the body's own material ("self") and that which is foreign ("nonself").

B lymphocytes: White blood cells that trigger the production of antibodies.

Bioavailability: The degree to which a nutrient or other substance becomes available for use in the body after ingestion or injection.

Carotenoids: Any of a group of red, yellow or orange pigments that are found in foods such as carrots, sweet potatoes and leafy green vegetables. The body converts these substances to vitamin A.

Carotid arteries: Arteries that bring blood from the heart to the brain via the neck.

Case control studies: Studies that compare people with a certain medical problem ("cases") with similar people who have not developed that medical problem ("controls").

Cataracts: Cloudings of the lens of the eye that obstruct vision.

Cell-mediated immunity: The type of immunity granted by T lymphocytes that helps the body resist infection.

Cerebrovascular: Dealing with the brain and the blood vessels.

Cholesterol: A white, waxy substance found naturally throughout the body, belonging to a class of compounds called sterols. Cholesterol is needed by the body to make hormones, vitamin D and bile acids and to build cells.

Coronary-artery disease: Atherosclerosis (blockage) of the coronary arteries, the spaghetti-size arteries that deliver blood to the heart.

Cystic fibrosis: An inherited disorder of glands that secrete through ducts; cystic fibrosis increases the risk of vitamin E deficiency.

Daily Value: See **Reference Daily Intake (RDI)**.

Diabetes: A disease resulting from the body's inability to produce or use insulin, resulting in high blood sugar levels.

Dietary Reference Intakes (DRIs): Dietary recommendations made by the National Academy of Sciences. These recommendations, which include four categories of reference intakes, are intended to replace the Recommended Dietary Allowances. They include Recommended Dietary Allowances, Adequate Intakes, Estimated Average Requirements and Tolerable Upper Intake Levels.

DRIs: See **Dietary Reference Intakes (DRIs)**.

Endothelium: A layer of cells that lines and protects the inner surfaces of blood vessels.

Epidemiologic studies: Studies to determine the distribution and causes of various health problems. These studies involve surveillance, observation, hypothesis-testing and experimentation.

Epilepsy: A group of nervous system disorders characterized by seizures, sensory disorders, abnormal behavior and/or blackouts.

Fat soluble: A type of vitamin that can be stored in the body for a long period of time and requires some fat for absorption; vitamin E is fat soluble.

Fibrocystic breast disease: Harmless lumps, or cysts, in the breast that can increase the risk of breast cancer.

Foam cells: Large, foamy-looking immune cells—macrophages—after they have eaten lots of cholesterol. Foam cells contribute to the development of atherosclerotic plaque.

Free radicals: Molecular fragments that attempt to steal electrons from other molecules. Free radicals have been linked to a number of chronic diseases, including heart disease and cancer.

Gamma-tocopherol: A form of vitamin E prevalent in corn and soybean oils.

HDL: See **High-density lipoprotein (HDL).**

Hemochromatosis: A disease in which iron builds up in the body, often affecting the liver.

Hemorrhagic stroke: A type of stroke caused by the rupture or leakage of blood vessels in or on the brain.

Hepatitis: Inflammation of the liver; hepatitis can be caused by a bacterial or a viral infection.

High-density lipoprotein (HDL): The so-called good cholesterol that helps to escort cholesterol from the body. High levels are linked with reduced risk of heart disease.

Humoral immunity: The form of immunity provided by the development and presence of antibodies.

Huntington's disease: A rare, inherited disease characterized by progressive dementia and irregular, involuntary movements of the limbs and facial muscles.

Immune response: The manner in which the immune system protects the body from disease. There are two types of immune response: humoral and cell-mediated.

Immune system: A complex system that protects the body from disease organisms and other foreign bodies; includes the humoral immune response and the cell-mediated immune response.

Insulin: A hormone produced in the pancreas that enables the body to use sugar for energy.

Interleukin-1: A beneficial immune system mediator that activates T cells and macrophages.

Interleukin-2: A beneficial immune system mediator that activates T cells.

Intermittent claudication: Periodic cramping pains in the calves caused by poor circulation of blood in the legs.

International units (I.U.): Arbitrary units of measurement that allow the various forms of certain vitamins—notably E and A—to be compared with one another.

Ischemic stroke: A type of stroke caused by insufficient blood flow to the brain.

I.U.: See **International units (I.U.)**.

LDL: See **Low-density lipoprotein (LDL)**.

Leukocytes: White blood cells.

Lipid peroxidation: Oxidation of fats, or lipids, in the body; an early stage in the development of atherosclerotic plaque.

Low-density lipoprotein (LDL): The so-called bad cholesterol. High levels of LDL cholesterol have been linked with increased risk of heart disease.

Lymphokines: Chemicals produced and released by T lymphocytes that attract phagocytes to the site of an infection or inflammation.

Macrophages: Large immune cells that can surround and digest foreign substances in the body.

Mediators: Chemicals that mediate, or act on, various components of the immune system; these chemicals provoke inflammation and cause the symptoms of allergic reactions.

Megadoses: Doses that exceed recommendations; scientifically, doses that are 10 times the RDA or more.

Mineral: A nonorganic compound, one that doesn't contain carbon and does not originate from living organisms.

Nitrosamines: Potentially carcinogenic substances formed in the digestive tract from nitrates and nitrites.

Nutrients: Substances used by the body that must be supplied from foods consumed. The six classes of nutrients are water, proteins, carbohydrates, fats, minerals and vitamins.

Oxidation: A chemical process in which a molecule combines with oxygen and loses electrons. Antioxidant nutrients such as vitamins C and E help control oxidation.

Pancreatitis: Swelling of the pancreas, which helps the body metabolize fat; pancreatitis can lead to vitamin E deficiency.

Parkinson's disease: A progressive disorder of the central nervous system that causes a deficiency of the neurotransmitter dopamine; its symptoms include tremors, stiffness in the limbs and joints, speech impediments, difficulty initiating physical movement and dementia.

Phagocytes: Immune cells that engulf and digest organisms and cell waste; macrophages are a type of phagocyte.

Placebo: An inactive substance.

Placebo-controlled study: A study in which the effectiveness of a treatment is compared with the effectiveness of a placebo, or inactive, substance.

Plaque: A deposit of fatty (and other) substances in the inner lining of the artery wall characteristic of atherosclerosis.

Plasma: The fluid portion of blood.

Platelets: Small, disk-shaped structures involved in blood coagulation.

Polyps: Masses of tissue that bulge or project outward or upward from the normal surface level.

Pro-oxidant: Promoting oxidation.

Prostaglandin E_2: A hormonelike fatty acid that suppresses the production of beneficial immune system mediators.

Protein kinase C: An enzyme that stimulates the production of smooth muscle cells, contributing to the development of scar tissue.

RDA: See **Recommended Dietary Allowance (RDA)**.

RDI: See **Reference Daily Intake (RDI)**.

Recommended Dietary Allowance (RDA): The level of intake of essential nutrients that, on the basis of scientific knowledge, is judged by the National Academy of Sciences' Food and Nutrition Board to be adequate to meet the known nutrient needs of practically all healthy persons.

Reference Daily Intake (RDI): The recommended level of nutrient intake per day that the U.S. Food and Drug Administration has approved for use on food labels; also called the Daily Value.

Retinopathy of prematurity (ROP): A condition developed by some premature infants in which abnormal blood vessels and scar tissue grow over the retina, affecting vision.

Rheumatoid arthritis: A chronic disease with inflammatory changes occurring throughout the body's connective tissues.

ROP: See **Retinopathy of prematurity (ROP)**.

Sprue: A long-term disorder caused by poor absorption of digested food in the small intestine that can lead to vitamin E deficiency.

Stroke: A sudden loss of function of part of the brain due to an interference in blood supply.

Supplements: Vitamins, minerals and other nutrients taken either alone or in combination to "supplement" the amount received through the diet.

T lymphocytes: White blood cells responsible for cell-mediated immunity.

Tardive dyskinesia: A condition in which the muscles of the face, limbs and trunk engage in repetitious, involuntary movements; a side effect of long-term use of psychoactive drugs.

TE: See **Tocopherol equivalents (TE)**.

Thrombophlebitis: Swelling of a vein along with the formation of a clot that frequently occurs as a result of an increased tendency of the blood to clot.

Thymus: A gland that is part of the immune system; T lymphocytes mature here.

Tocopherol equivalents (TE): Arbitrary units of measurement that enable the different forms of vitamin E to be compared with one another. One TE or one milligram TE is equal to 1.49 international units.

Tocopherols: Compounds that exhibit vitamin E activity; there are four tocopherols—alpha, beta, delta and gamma.

Tocotrienols: Compounds that exhibit vitamin E activity.

Triglycerides: Fatty compounds found in the blood.

Vasodilators: Substances that cause blood vessels to dilate, improving blood flow.

Vitamin E: A fat-soluble, light yellow oil with antioxidant properties; any of eight tocopherols or tocotrienols.

Vitamin E quinone: A vitamin E derivative with anticoagulant properties.

Vitamins: Organic components of food found to be essential in small quantities for normal human metabolism, growth and physical well-being.

Water soluble: Able to be dissolved in water. The water-soluble vitamins—the B vitamins and vitamin C—are not stored in the body but are quickly excreted.

Wilson's disease: A rare, inherited disorder in which copper accumulates in the liver and is then released and taken up into other parts of the body.

INDEX

A

Acquired immunodeficiency syndrome (AIDS). *See* AIDS
Aging
  immune system effects, 56
  vitamin E effects, 53, 54, 78
AIDS, vitamin E effects, 53
Alcohol, effects, 100
Allergic skin reactions, vitamin E, 80
Alpha-tocopherol
  defined, 12, 113
  effects, 105
Alpha-tocopheroxyl radical, defined, 35, 113
Alzheimer's disease
  defined, 21, 113
  selegiline effects, 69
  vitamin E effects, 11, 21, 65, 66, 68-71
Anemia
  defined, 16, 113
  hemolytic, causes, 84, 100
Angina
  defined, 25, 113
  vitamin E effects, 25, 42-43
Antibodies, defined, 49, 113
Anticoagulants
  defined, 19, 113
  effects, 19, 48, 101-102
Antigens, defined, 49, 113
Antioxidant, defined, 12-13, 113
Arthritis, rheumatoid
  defined, 84, 119
  vitamin E effects, 84, 87
Aspirin, stroke prevention, 47
Asthma
  vitamin C effects, 74-75
  vitamin E effects, 74-75
Atherosclerosis
  causes, 29-30
  defined, 28, 114
  vitamin E effects, 28-41, 83-84
Autoimmune diseases, defined, 56, 114

B

B cells. *See* B lymphocytes
B lymphocytes, defined, 49, 114
Bacterial infections, effects, 29
Bioavailability, defined, 106, 114
Blood clots, vitamin E effects, 39-42
Blood flow, vitamin E effects, 41-43, 48
Blood pressure, effects, 29
Blood vessels
  vitamin C effects, 38-39
  vitamin E effects, 38-39

Breast cancer, vitamin E effects, 60-61, 64
Breast-feeding, vitamin E, Recommended Dietary Allowances (RDAs), 94

C

Cancer
  breast, vitamin E effects, 60-61, 64
  colon, vitamin E effects, 61-62
  generally, prevention
    revised Recommended Dietary Allowances (RDAs), 18-19
    vitamin E effects, 52, 56-57
  lung
    beta carotene effects, 57-58
    vitamin A effects, 59-60
    vitamin C effects, 59-60
    vitamin E effects, 57-60, 63
  oral
    carotenoids effects, 62
    vitamin E effects, 62
  promotion, vitamin E effects, 63-64
  prostate, vitamin E effects, 62-63
  rectal, vitamin E effects, 61-62
  skin, vitamin E effects, 78-79
  stomach
    beta carotene effects, 62-63
    selenium effects, 62-63
    vitamin E effects, 62-63
  treatment
    beta carotene effects, 63
    vitamin A effects, 63
    vitamin C effects, 63
    vitamin E effects, 63
  vitamin E effects, 11, 21, 64-65, 90
Carotenoids
  defined, 62, 114
  oral cancer, 62
Carotid arteries, defined, 29, 114
Case control studies, defined, 25, 114

Cataracts
  defined, 21, 114
  protection, vitamin E effects, 21
  vitamin E effects, 75-77
Cell-mediated immunity, defined, 50, 114
Cerebrovascular, defined, 47, 114
Children/infants
  epilepsy, vitamin E effects, 68
  retinopathy of prematurity (ROP), vitamin E effects, 77
  vitamin E, Recommended Dietary Allowances (RDAs), 94
  vitamin E deficiencies
    causes, 98
    signs, 96
Cholesterol
  defined, 28, 114
  medications, vitamin E interactions, 102
  vitamin E effects, 32-36
Cirrhosis, liver, effects, 84, 88
Colestid, vitamin E interactions, 102
Colon cancer, vitamin E effects, 61-62
Contraception, oral, vitamin E interactions, 102
Coronary-artery disease
  defined, 28, 114
  vitamin E effects, 28
Coumadin. *See* Warfarin
Cystic fibrosis
  defined, 17, 115
  effects, 17, 23, 66, 84, 98

D

Daily Value. *See* Reference Daily Intake (RDI)
Danazol, effects, 86
Danocrine. *See* Danazol
Deprenyl. *See* Selegiline
Diabetes
  defined, 21, 115

INDEX

effects, 41
vitamin E effects, 21, 81-84, 90
Diarrhea, causes, 19
Diet, low-fat, effects, 98
Dietary Reference Intakes (DRIs)
defined, 18, 115
vitamin E, 18, 96
dl-Alpha-tocopherol nicotinate, effects, 47
Doxorubicin, effects on wound healing, 80
DRIs. *See* Dietary Reference Intakes (DRIs)
Drug interactions, vitamin E, 19, 101-102

E

Elderly, vitamin E effects, 52, 54-56
Endothelial function, vitamin E effects, 28-29, 37-39, 48
Endothelium, defined, 28-29, 115
Epidemiologic studies, defined, 23, 115
Epilepsy
defined, 66, 115
vitamin E effects, 66, 68
Exercise
effects, 100
vitamin E effects, 84-85
Eye conditions, vitamin E effects, 75-77

F

Fainting, causes, 19
Fat
absorption problems, 17, 23, 66, 98, 102
polyunsaturated, effects, 99
Fat soluble, defined, 12, 115
Fertility, vitamin E effects, 88-89
Fibrocystic breast disease
defined, 86, 115
vitamin E effects, 86

Flatulence, causes, 19
Foam cells, defined, 30, 115
Free radicals
defined, 13, 116
formation, 30

G

Gamma-tocopherol
defined, 99, 116
effects, 99, 105

H

HDL. *See* High-density lipoprotein (HDL)
Headache, causes, 19
Heart attack, vitamin E effects, 43-44
Heart disease
revised Recommended Dietary Allowance (RDA), 18-19
vitamin C effects, 23-24
vitamin E effects, 11, 21, 22-23, 23-24, 43-44, 82-84, 90
Heart palpitations, causes, 19
Hemochromatosis
defined, 88, 116
vitamin E effects, 88
Hemorrhagic stroke
defined, 47, 116
vitamin E effects, 47-48
Hepatitis
defined, 88, 116
vitamin E effects, 88
High-density lipoprotein (HDL), defined, 36, 116
Hormone replacement therapy, vitamin E interactions, 102
Humoral immunity, defined, 49, 116
Huntington's disease
defined, 66, 116
vitamin E effects, 66, 67
Hypersensitivity pneumonitis, vitamin E effects, 74

I

Illness, effects, 23
Immune response
  defined, 21, 50-51, 116
  vitamin E effects, 21, 22, 49-56
Immune system
  components, 49-53
  defined, 14, 116
Immunoglobulin G, vitamin E effects, 52
Influenza, vitamin E effects, 53-54
Insulin
  defined, 81, 116
  vitamin E effects, 82-83
Interleukin-1
  defined, 52, 116
  vitamin C effects, 52
  vitamin E effects, 52
Interleukin-2
  defined, 52, 117
  vitamin E effects, 52
Intermittent claudication
  defined, 42, 117
  vitamin E effects, 42
International units (I.U.), defined, 17, 58, 95, 117
Ischemic stroke, defined, 46, 117
I.U. See International units (I.U.)

L

Laxatives, vitamin E interactions, 102
LDL. See Low-density lipoprotein (LDL)
Leukocytes, defined, 28, 117
Leukoplakia
  beta carotene effects, 62
  vitamin E effects, 62
Lipid peroxidation
  defined, 13, 30, 117
Liver disease, chronic, effects, 17, 23, 66, 98
Liver function, vitamin E effects, 84, 87-88

Low-density lipoprotein (LDL)
  defined, 28, 117
  vitamin E effects, 28, 29, 30, 32-36, 48
Lung, protection, vitamin E effects, 21
Lung cancer
  beta carotene effects, 57-58
  vitamin A effects, 59-60
  vitamin C effects, 59-60
  vitamin E effects, 57-60, 63
Lung function, vitamin E effects, 72-75
Lupus, vitamin A, vitamin E, beta carotene levels, 87
Lymphokines, defined, 50, 117

M

Macrophages, defined, 30, 117
Mediators, defined, 50, 117
Megadoses, defined, 100-101, 117
Melanoma, vitamin E effects, 63
Mineral oil laxatives, vitamin E interactions, 102
Minerals
  defined, 15, 115
  selenium
    antioxidant effects, 15
    platelet function, 41
    stomach cancer, 62-63
    stroke prevention, 46-47
  supplements, 103-104
Muscle function, vitamin E effects, 84-85
Muscle soreness, vitamin E effects, 21

N

Nausea, causes, 19
Nervous system, vitamin E effects, 65-71
Nitrates
  defined, 65
  sources, 65

Nitrites
  defined, 65
  sources, 65
Nitrosamines
  defined, 64-65, 117
  effects, 64-65
Nutrient interactions, vitamin E, 102-103
Nutrients, defined, 11, 118

O

Oral cancer
  carotenoids effects, 62
  vitamin E effects, 62
Oral contraceptives, vitamin E interactions, 102
Osteoporosis, generally, prevention, revised Recommended Dietary Allowances (RDAs), 18-19
Oxidation, defined, 13, 118

P

Palpitations, causes, 19
Pancreatitis
  defined, 66, 118
  effects, 66, 84, 98
Parkinson's disease
  defined, 66, 118
  vitamin E effects, 66-67
Phagocytes, defined, 50, 118
Physicians, vitamin E supplement intake, 22-23
Placebo, defined, 28, 118
Placebo-controlled study, defined, 28, 118
Plaque, defined, 28, 118
Plasma, defined, 23, 118
Platelet, defined, 29, 118
Platelet function
  beta carotene effects, 41
  selenium effects, 41
  vitamin C effects, 41
  vitamin E effects, 39-42, 48

Pollutants, effects, 73, 100
Polyps, defined, 62, 118
Polyunsaturated fats, effects, 99
Pregnancy
  effects, 100
  vitamin E, Recommended Dietary Allowance (RDA), 94
Prematurity
  retinopathy of prematurity (ROP), vitamin E effects, 77
  vitamin E levels, 98
Premenstrual symptoms, vitamin E effects, 86
Pressure sores, vitamin E effects, 80
Pro-oxidant, defined, 34, 118
Pro-oxidant effects, vitamin E, 34-36, 63-64
Prostaglandin E_2, defined, 51, 118
Prostate cancer, vitamin E effects, 62-63
Protein kinase C, defined, 37, 118

Q

Questran, vitamin E interactions, 102

R

RDA. *See* Recommended Dietary Allowance (RDA)
RDI. *See* Reference Daily Intake (RDI)
Recommended Dietary Allowance (RDA)
  defined, 17, 119
  vitamin E, 17, 94-96
Rectal cancer, vitamin E effects, 61-62
Reference Daily Intake (RDI), defined, 18, 119
Research techniques, discrepancies, 89-91
Respiratory system, vitamin E effects, 72-75

Retinopathy of prematurity (ROP)
  defined, 77, 119
  vitamin E effects, 77
Rheumatoid arthritis
  defined, 84, 119
  vitamin E effects, 84, 87
ROP. See Retinopathy of prematurity (ROP)

S

Scars, vitamin E effects, 78, 79-80
Selegiline, Alzheimer's disease, 69
Skin, vitamin E effects, 78-81
Skin cancer, vitamin E effects, 78-79
Smoking
  effects, 29, 34, 57-58, 60, 72-73, 100
  vitamin E effects on lungs, 72-73
Smooth muscle cells, vitamin E effects, 37, 48
Sprue
  defined, 66, 119
  effects, 66, 84
Stomach cancer
  beta carotene effects, 62-63
  selenium effects, 62-63
  vitamin E effects, 62-63
Stress, effects, 72-73
Stroke
  defined, 21, 119
  hemorrhagic
    defined, 47, 116
    vitamin E effects, 47-48
  ischemic, defined, 46, 117
  protection, vitamin C effects, 21
  risk factors, 46
  vitamin E effects, 28, 46-48
Sunburn, vitamin E effects, 78-79
Supplements, defined, 11, 119

T

T cells. See T lymphocytes
T lymphocytes, defined, 50, 114
Tardive dyskinesia
  defined, 66, 119
  vitamin E effects, 66, 68
TE. See Tocopherol equivalents (TE)
Thrombophlebitis
  defined, 42, 120
  vitamin E effects, 42
Thymus gland, defined, 49, 120
Tocopherol equivalents (TE), defined, 17, 58, 95, 120
Tocopherols, defined, 11-12, 120
Tocopheryl sorbate, defined, 78
Tocotrienols, defined, 11-12, 120
Tolerable Upper Intake, defined, 19
Toxicity, vitamin E, 100-101
Transient ischemic attacks, defined, 47
Triad, effects on wound healing, 80
Triglycerides
  defined, 39, 120
  vitamin E effects, 82
Tumor necrosis factor alpha
  vitamin C effects, 52
  vitamin E effects, 52

U

Ultraviolet radiation, vitamin E effects, 78-79

V

Vasodilators, defined, 38, 120
Viral infections, effects, 29
Vitamin E quinone, defined, 40, 120

Vitamins
 beta carotene
  antioxidant effects, 15
  atherosclerosis, 33-34
  cancer treatment, 63
  effects on vitamin E, 103
  lung cancer, 57-58
  lupus, 87
  platelet function, 41
  stomach cancer, 62-63
  stroke prevention, 46-47
  defined, 12, 120
  measurements
   international units (I.U.), 17-18, 58, 95
   tocopherol equivalents (TE), 17-18, 58, 95
  multivitamins, vitamin E supplements vs., 55, 103-104
  nicotinic acid, effects, 47
  supplements, defined, 11, 119
 vitamin A
  cancer treatment, 63
  lung cancer, 59-60
  lupus, 87
  measurement units, 17
 vitamin C
  antioxidant effects, 15
  asthma, 74-75
  atherosclerosis, 33-34
  blood vessels, 38-39
  cancer treatment, 63
  effects on vitamin E, 35, 99-100, 102-103
  heart disease protection, 23-24
  immune system, 52
  lung cancer, 59-60
  platelet function, 41
  supplement popularity, 11
 vitamin E
  aging, 53, 54
  AIDS, 53
  Alzheimer's disease, 11, 21, 65, 66, 68-71
  angina, 25, 42-43
  anticoagulant effects, 19, 48, 101-102
  antioxidant role, 12-15
  asthma, 74-75
  atherosclerosis, 28-41, 30-32, 33-34, 40-41, 83-84
  blood clots, 39-42
  blood flow, 41-43, 48
  blood vessels, 37-39
  breast cancer, 60-61, 64
  cancer prevention, 52, 56-57
  cancer promotion, 63-64
  cancer protection, 21, 64-65, 90
  cancer risk, 57-63
  cancer treatment, 63, 63-65
  cataracts, 21, 75-77
  cholesterol, 32-36
  colon cancer, 61-62
  coronary-artery disease, 28
  deficiencies
   causes, 17, 23, 66, 84, 98
   immune system effects, 51-52
   nervous system effects, 65-66
   signs, 16-17, 96
  defined, 11, 120
  diabetes, 21, 81-84, 90
  Dietary Reference Intakes (DRIs), 18, 96
  dietary sources, 20, 95, 98, 99, 102, 109-111
  dosage
   discrepancies, 97-100
   recommended, 19
  drug interactions, 19, 101-102
  effects, generally, 11
  endothelial function, 28-29, 37-39, 48
  epilepsy, 66, 68
  fertility, 88-89
  fibrocystic breast disease, 86
  forms, 11-12
  heart attack prevention, 43-44
  heart disease protection, 11, 21, 22-28, 43-45, 82-84, 90

hemorrhagic stroke, 47-48
hepatitis, 88
high doses, side effects, 19
Huntington's disease, 66, 67
hypersensitivity pneumonitis, 74
immune response, 21, 22, 49-56
influenza, 53-54
interaction with beta carotene, 103
interaction with vitamin C, 35, 99-100, 102-103
intermittent claudication, 42
liver function, 84, 87-88
low-density lipoprotein (LDL) levels, 28, 29, 30, 32-36, 48
lung cancer, 57-60, 63
lung function, 72-75
lung protection, 21
lupus, 87
megadoses
  defined, 100-101, 117
  side effects, 19
melanoma, 63
muscle function, 84-85
muscle soreness, 21
nervous system, 65-71
nutrient interactions, 102-103
oral cancer, 62
Parkinson's disease, 66-67
physicians' supplement intake, 22-23
platelet function, 39-42, 48
premenstrual symptoms, 86
primary function, 12
pro-oxidant effects, 34-36, 63-64
prostate cancer, 62-63
Recommended Dietary Allowances (RDAs), 17, 94-96
rectal cancer, 61-62
respiratory system, 72-75
retinopathy of prematurity (ROP), 77
rheumatoid arthritis, 84, 87
role in body functions, 12-16
skin, 78-81
smooth muscle cells, 37, 48
stomach cancer, 62-63
stroke protection, 21, 28, 46-48
supplements
  absorption, 108-109
  forms, 103-109
  natural vs. synthetic, 105-107
  popularity, 11
  storage, 109
  vs. multivitamins, 55, 103-104
tardive dyskinesia, 66, 68
thrombophlebitis, 42
toxicity, 100-101
white blood cells, 36, 48
wound healing, 78, 79-81
vitamin K deficiency, 48, 101-102

W

Warfarin, vitamin E interactions, 19, 101-102
Water soluble, defined, 12, 120
White blood cells, vitamin E effects, 36, 48
Wilson's disease, defined, 88, 120
Wound healing, vitamin E effects, 78, 79-80
Wrinkles, vitamin E effects, 78